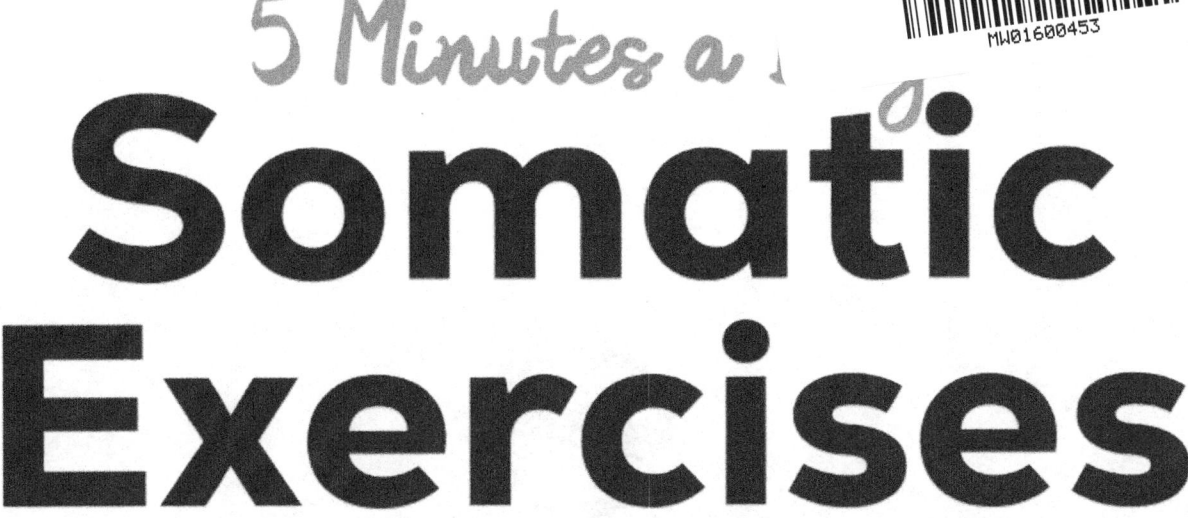

5 Minutes a Day
Somatic Exercises
for Nervous System Regulation

TARA ZEN

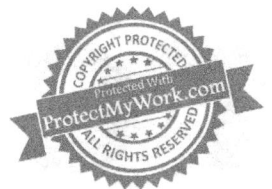

TABLE OF CONTENTS

Video Course and Tracking Journal Included

Before you start! I've got something special for you: a special bonus package that complements and expands on the exercises. This bonus package that I've prepared for you is designed to support your ongoing practice and help you integrate somatic awareness into your daily life.

To access the package, simply use your smartphone's camera to scan the QR code below and you'll be directed to a secure download page where you will receive a google drive link to the workbook and a vimeo link for a more visual interpretation of the exercises. What's included in your bonus package:

- A video course for the somatic exercises covered in the book.
- A tracking journal integrating what you've learned into your daily routine and much more!

This content is here to support you as you continue to explore, grow, and deepen your connection with your body's wisdom.

Happy exploring, and may your somatic journey be rich and rewarding!

INTRODUCTION

You've heard it before: "Listen to your body." But what does that really mean to you?

Take a moment. Close your eyes, if you will. What comes to mind when you think about listening to your body? Maybe you see yourself paying attention to hunger pangs, noticing a tight neck after a long day at the computer, or feeling your heart race before a big presentation; these are all valid interpretations, but there's so much more to discover.

You're probably juggling a million responsibilities as someone with a demanding career or a full life. Your to-do list never seems to end; between work deadlines, family obligations, and trying to maintain some semblance of social life, the idea of "listening to your body" is yet another task you don't have time for, and I get it. I've been there, too, and I've learned a humbling lesson: you can't rush through life and expect your nervous system to relax on command.

Think about it: how often do you find yourself racing from one task to the next, only to collapse on the couch at the end of the day, wondering why you can't seem to unwind? Your body doesn't have an on/off switch for stress. It needs time, attention, and the right tools to find balance.

Somatic therapy, in these instances, reminds us that we are living with our bodies, not just in them, but let me be clear: this isn't psychotherapy. Somatic therapy's primary intent is to awaken you to the inherent wisdom carried in your body. It gives you the tools you need to access this wisdom—a wisdom that's been there all along, waiting for you to tune in. This book isn't about adding more to your already full plate. It's about giving you practical, science-backed tools that fit into your busy life. Through these mindful, body-based practices, you'll learn to tap into your body's innate wisdom and its ability to regulate your nervous system.

These techniques are designed for real life— your life and don't require hours of your time or a complete overhaul of your schedule. Many can be done in just a few minutes, seamlessly integrated into your daily routine. Whether you're sitting at your desk, waiting in line at the grocery store, or lying in bed unable to sleep, these exercises are there for you.

You'll learn how your body and mind are connected, why this matters for your mental health, and, most importantly, how to use this knowledge to your advantage. You'll learn simple yet powerful exercises that can help you reduce stress, manage anxiety, and cultivate a greater sense of well-being, all while honoring the demands of your busy life.

Chapter 1: What is Somatic Exercise

The human body is not an instrument to be used but a realm of one's being to be experienced, explored, enriched, and, thereby, educated—
Thomas Hannah

Buddhists see the body as a tool of liberation. In their traditions, the body is an integral part of our journey toward enlightenment and inner peace. This perspective invites us to consider our bodies not as separate entities to be controlled or ignored but as wise companions on our path to well-being. In many ways, modern somatic practices echo this ancient understanding; they remind us that our bodies hold deep wisdom accumulated through every experience we've ever had. Each tension, each breath, each subtle movement tells a story—if only we learn to listen.

So many of us, however, have lost touch with this bodily wisdom. We push through fatigue, ignore stress signals, and disconnect from physical sensations in our rush to meet the next deadline or obligation. We've become skilled at overriding our body's messages, sometimes to our own detriment. Somatic exercises offer a bridge back to our bodies, a way to reconnect with the physical wisdom we've always possessed but perhaps forgotten how to access.

The term 'somatic' comes from the Greek word 'soma', meaning 'living body.' In the context of therapy and exercise, somatic exercises refer to approaches that engage the whole self—body, mind, and spirit. By extension, somatic exercises work on the principle that the mind and body are inextricably linked. What affects one inevitably influences the other. Somatic exercises, therefore, are practices that use the body as a gateway to overall well-being. They focus on developing body awareness, releasing tension, and learning to regulate the nervous system through mindful movement and breathing and can range from simple breathing techniques to more complex movement patterns. They might involve gentle stretches, focused attention on bodily sensations, or exploration of how emotions manifest physically. The key is that they all aim to increase your ability to sense, feel, and respond to what's happening in your body in the present moment.

When you engage in somatic exercises, you're not just working out—you're working in. You're developing a keener sense of your internal landscape, learning to recognize and respond to stress signals earlier, and cultivating a deeper sense of embodiment in your daily life.

So, as we work through this chapter, I want you to keep the Buddhist perspective we started with in mind: that your body is not just a vehicle for your mind but a profound tool for transformation and liberation. When you listen to and work with your body, you're replenishing the resources that sustain you and are life-giving, which equip you with greater peace, resilience, and well-being in all aspects of your life.

The Science Behind Somatic Exercises

To be able to change how we feel, we need to become more familiar with our internal landscapes. In his groundbreaking book "The Body Keeps the Score," psychiatrist Bessel van der Kolk emphasizes that trauma and stress are not just mental states but physical experiences stored within our bodies. When we engage with our bodily sensations, movements, and internal rhythms, we rewire our nervous systems and create lasting changes in our emotional and mental well-being.

The effectiveness of somatic exercises is rooted in neuroplasticity, the brain's ability to form new neural connections throughout life. Consistent body awareness and mindful movement practice help create new neural pathways that override old stress and reactivity patterns, replacing them with calmer, more regulated responses. Studies have shown that regular engagement in mindfulness and body-based practices can lead to changes in brain structure, particularly in areas associated with emotional regulation, self-awareness, and stress response.

Somatic exercises also work directly with the autonomic nervous system, which controls our fight-flight-freeze responses; it guides the body through specific movements and breathing patterns, which can help shift the nervous system from a state of high alert (sympathetic activation) to a state of rest and digest (parasympathetic activation). This shift is necessary for managing stress and anxiety, as it allows the body to move out of survival mode and into a state where healing, recovery, and rational thinking can occur. It equips us to handle life's challenges without becoming overwhelmed or shutting down.

Benefits of Somatic Exercises for Stress and Anxiety

Our way of being touches everyone around us; how we show up in our relationships, work, and the world around us all begins with what is going on in our nervous systems. When we're constantly stressed or anxious, it affects our internal experience and how we interact with others and navigate our daily lives.

At their core, somatic exercises enhance body awareness and improve the mind-body connection, and this increased awareness allows you to recognize the early signs of stress or anxiety, enabling you to intervene before these feelings escalate. Through gentle movements and focused attention, these exercises shift your nervous system from a state of high alert to a state of calm, building your capacity to handle stress; you become more resilient, able to bounce back more quickly from stressful events and maintain equilibrium in challenging situations.

Beyond these immediate benefits, regular practice cultivates a deeper, more compassionate relationship with yourself. The more attuned you are to your body and its needs, you naturally develop greater self-compassion and a stronger sense of agency over your well-being; this internal shift ripples outward, positively influencing how you engage with others and navigate the world around you—you're fostering a richer, more embodied sense of living, and do keep in mind: the goal isn't to eliminate stress and anxiety entirely, but to build your capacity to move through these experiences with greater ease and resilience, ultimately improving the quality of your life and relationships.

The Principles of Somatic Exercises

A nervous system at ease is the foundation of well-being; the state where your body feels safest, your mind is at its clearest, and you can engage with life from a place of wholeness. Somatic exercises offer a path back to nervous system regulation and overall wellness. These exercises are built on several core principles that work together to promote physical and mental well-being. Let's unpack these principles in depth:

Mindfulness

Mindfulness is your ability to be present in the moment; it's observing your thoughts, feelings, and bodily sensations without judgment and cultivating a state of open awareness of your current experience. It is the foundation for all other practices as it helps you:

- Tune into your body's subtle cues and messages
- Notice thought patterns and emotional responses
- Develop a non-reactive stance towards your experiences
- Foster a deeper connection between mind and body

In practice, it might involve:

- Taking a few moments to notice your breath without trying to change it
- Scanning your body and noticing sensations without labeling them as good or bad
- Observing your thoughts and emotions as they arise, without getting caught up in their content

Body Awareness

This means having a keen sense of what's happening in your body and noticing tensions, movements, temperature changes, and other physical sensations. Enhanced body awareness allows you to recognize stress signals early and respond appropriately.

Developing body awareness includes:

- Recognizing areas of tension or ease in your body
- Noticing your posture and how it affects your mood
- Being aware of your breath patterns
- Sensing how different emotions manifest physically in your body

For example, you might notice that when you're anxious, your shoulders tense up, or when you're happy, there's a warmth in your chest. This awareness can serve as an early warning system for stress and a guide for self-regulation.

Gentle Movement

Somatic exercises often involve slow, deliberate movements. These aren't about pushing your body to its limits but rather about exploring your body's current capabilities and boundaries. Gentle movement helps release tension, improve flexibility, and increase your range of movement; this involves:

- Moving slowly and with intention
- Staying within a comfortable range of motion
- Paying attention to the quality of movement rather than quantity
- Using breath to support movement

For instance, a gentle movement exercise might involve slowly rolling your shoulders while paying attention to any sensations that arise or mindfully walking while focusing on the feeling of your feet touching the ground.

Resourcing

Resourcing is how skilled you are at self-regulation and your ability to utilize positive coping mechanisms. In essence, it's about having an anchor that helps stabilize you when feeling dysregulated. Think of it as your personal toolkit for wellness, always at your disposal when you need to find balance.

Resources can be either external or internal:

- External resources are people, places, pets, or activities that feel safe and comforting. It might be the memory of a supportive friend, a favorite peaceful location, the soothing presence of a pet, or an engaging hobby that brings you joy.
- Internal resources are positive sensations in the body or emotional states that bring a sense of calm and stability. This could be the feeling of your feet firmly planted on the ground, a sense of warmth in your chest, or the memory of a time when you felt confident and capable.

In somatic practice, you learn to identify and cultivate these resources, making them more readily available when needed. The goal is to create a sense of support and stability you can access even in challenging moments.

Tracking

Tracking in somatic exercises refers to becoming more aware of our body's sensations and physiological responses. It's a practice of paying close attention to physical sensations, such as tension, heartbeat, and breath, without reacting to them with panic, fear, worry, judgment, or attempting to change them.

The key to effective tracking is cultivating a stance of curious observation. You're not trying to change anything; you're simply noticing what's happening in your body from moment to moment. This might involve:

- Scanning your body and noticing areas of tension or ease
- Observing the rhythm and depth of your breath
- Paying attention to subtle shifts in sensation, like changes in temperature or tingling
- Noticing how emotions manifest physically in your body

An important aspect of tracking is reminding yourself that these sensations are safe and not putting you in any real danger. This is especially crucial when working with uncomfortable or intense sensations. The goal is to view these sensations without fear and judgment, helping to calm your nervous system and provide relief in the long term when these sensations arise.

Containment

Containment is the ability to tolerate negative sensations and emotions without feeling out of control or reacting in an impulsive manner. It's having the capacity to stay present with our experiences and feelings, holding them in a way that they don't overwhelm or frighten us. This container is flexible enough to allow you to feel your emotions fully, but strong enough to prevent those emotions from spilling over into reactive behaviors.

Practicing containment involves:

1. Recognizing and acknowledging your emotions and sensations

2. Creating a sense of boundary around your experience

3. Regulating the intensity of the experience by focusing on present-moment sensations

4. Using grounding techniques to maintain a sense of stability

Containment doesn't mean suppressing or ignoring difficult emotions. Instead, it's about creating a safe space to experience them without being overwhelmed. This skill allows you to process emotions more effectively and respond to challenging situations with greater calm and intention.

All of these principles don't work in isolation, but rather in concert, each supporting and enhancing the others. For instance, mindfulness supports body awareness, allowing for more intentional gentle movement. They guide you towards a state where your nervous system can find ease, respond to life's challenges with flexibility and grace, and experience a deeper sense of embodiment in your daily life.

Chapter 2: Getting Started With Somatic Exercises

Your body is the ground metaphor of your life, the expression of your existence—Gabrielle Roth

They say that the more you move, the more you understand your body, however, this isn't just about movement—it's about awareness. It's about tuning into the subtle language of your body, a language that's been speaking to you all along.

Think about the last time you felt a knot of tension in your shoulders or a flutter of excitement in your stomach. These sensations are more than just physical experiences—they're your body's way of communicating. Somatic exercise teaches us to listen to these messages, to understand them, and to respond in ways that promote balance and well-being.

We're going to learn how to begin this dialogue with your body. We'll introduce gentle movements and awareness practices that are accessible to everyone, regardless of fitness level or physical ability. The goal isn't to achieve perfect form or push physical limits. Instead, it's about cultivating a deeper connection with yourself, learning to recognize and respond to your body's needs, and discovering the wealth of information your physical self holds. As we proceed, approach each exercise with curiosity and patience. Your body has a unique story to tell—one that's been shaped by your individual experiences, challenges, and triumphs. Now is the time to listen.

Preparing Your Space and Mind

The human mind thrives on beauty; that's why we crave aesthetically pleasing surroundings. This innate desire for beauty is deeply connected to our sense of well-being and our ability to relax and focus. When we create a space that feels beautiful and peaceful to us, we set the stage for a more effective practice of somatic exercises.

Your practice space is a physical representation of your commitment to self-care and inner exploration. It doesn't need to be large or elaborately decorated. What matters is that it feels welcoming and calming to you. This might mean clearing a corner of your bedroom, setting up a small altar with meaningful objects, or simply choosing a spot near a window where natural light can filter in. The key is to create an environment that signals to your mind and body that it's time to slow down, turn inward, and listen to the wisdom your body holds. When your surroundings support your practice, you'll find it easier to transition from the busyness of daily life into a state of mindful awareness, ready to engage fully with your somatic exercises.

Tips for Selecting and Organizing Your Practice Space

When choosing and setting up your space for somatic exercises, consider the following tips:

- **Choose a quiet location:** Select a spot where you're least likely to be disturbed. This could be a spare room, a corner of your bedroom, or even a peaceful outdoor space when weather permits.

- **Ensure adequate space:** You'll need enough room to lie down comfortably and move your arms and legs freely. A space about the size of a yoga mat is usually sufficient.

- **Optimize comfort:** The floor should be comfortable for lying down. Use a yoga mat, blanket, or carpet to provide cushioning.

- **Control the temperature:** Ensure the space is neither too hot nor too cold. You want to be comfortable enough to relax without being distracted by temperature.

- **Manage lighting:** Natural light is ideal, but if that's not possible, opt for soft, warm lighting. Harsh overhead lights can be distracting and make it harder to relax.

- **Minimize visual clutter:** A cluttered space can lead to a cluttered mind. Keep the area tidy and free from distractions.

- **Incorporate calming elements:** Consider adding plants, a small fountain, or artwork that you find soothing. These can help create a more relaxing atmosphere.

- **Have props ready:** Keep any props you might need (like pillows, blankets, or bolsters) nearby so you don't have to interrupt your practice to fetch them.

- **Create a scent-scape:** If you enjoy aromatherapy, consider using essential oils or incense to create a pleasant, calming scent in your practice space.

- **Set boundaries:** If you live with others, communicate the importance of your practice time and space. Ask for their support in maintaining a quiet environment during your practice.

- **Make it personal:** Add elements that are meaningful to you—perhaps a special photograph, an inspiring quote, or a small memento that helps you feel grounded and centered.

Essential Equipment and Attire

The tools that you use will determine the overall quality of your practice, and what I mean by this is that the right equipment and attire can significantly enhance your somatic experience. However, it's important to note that "right" doesn't necessarily mean expensive or elaborate. In somatic practice, simplicity often reigns supreme.

The tools for somatic therapy aren't complex machines or high-tech gadgets, just items that support your body, facilitate movement, and enhance your awareness. The goal is to create an environment and use tools that allow you to tune into your body's sensations without distraction or discomfort.

Your attire, too, plays a crucial role. The clothes you wear during your practice should allow for free movement and deep breathing, enabling you to focus on the subtle shifts and sensations in your body rather than on restrictive or uncomfortable clothing. Remember, the essence of somatic practice is about connecting with your body, and your equipment and attire should serve to facilitate this connection, not hinder it.

Essential Equipment and Attire for Somatic Practice

Comfortable Mat: A yoga or exercise mat provides cushioning and defines your practice space. Choose one that's thick enough for comfort but firm enough for stability.

1. **Comfortable Mat:** A yoga or exercise mat provides cushioning and defines your practice space. Choose one that's thick enough for comfort but firm enough for stability.
2. **Loose, Breathable Clothing:** Opt for soft, stretchy fabrics that allow for free movement. Examples include:
   - Loose-fitting T-shirts or tank tops
   - Comfortable pants or shorts
   - Breathable, stretchy leggings
3. **Blanket or Throw:** Useful for extra warmth or cushioning during floor exercises.
4. **Pillows or Bolsters:** These support different body parts during various exercises, enhancing comfort and alignment.
5. **Small Towel:** Handy for wiping away sweat or providing extra cushioning when

needed.

6. **Water Bottle:** Staying hydrated is important, especially if you're doing more active somatic exercises.

7. **Journal and Pen:** For recording insights, sensations, or progress after your practice.

8. **Timer or Clock:** To keep track of time during timed exercises without constantly checking your phone.

9. **Foam Roller:** Optional but beneficial for self-massage and releasing muscle tension.

10. **Therapy Balls:** Small, firm balls (like tennis balls) can be used for targeted pressure and release work.

11. **Eye Pillow:** Useful for relaxation exercises or to block out light during lying-down practices.

12. **Socks or Warm Footwear:** To keep feet warm during less active exercises.

You don't need all of these items to start. Have the basics first—comfortable clothing and a mat—and gradually add other items as you develop your practice and discover what works best for you.

Recommendations for Selecting Yoga Mats and Props

When choosing equipment for your somatic practice, quality and comfort are key. Here are some recommendations to guide your selection:

Yoga Mats

1. **Thickness:** For somatic work, opt for a mat between 4-6mm thick. This provides enough cushioning for comfort during floor work without being too soft for standing exercises.

2. **Material:** Look for mats made from eco-friendly materials like natural rubber, jute, or cork. These offer good grip and are environmentally sustainable.

3. **Texture:** Choose a mat with a slightly textured surface for better grip, especially if you tend to sweat.

4. **Size:** Standard mats (68" x 24") work well for most people, but if you're taller, consider a longer mat (72" or 74").

5. **Durability:** Invest in a high-quality mat that will last. Brands like Manduka, Jade, and Lululemon are known for their durability.

Props

When possible, try out equipment before purchasing. Many yoga and wellness stores allow you to test mats and props. This hands-on experience can help you find the items that feel best for your unique body and practice.

1. **Bolsters:**
   - Choose a firm bolster that's at least 24" long for versatile support.
   - Look for removable, washable covers for easy cleaning.

2. **Blankets:**
   - Mexican yoga blankets are ideal due to their firmness and versatility.
   - Choose 100% cotton for breathability and easy care.

3. **Blocks:**
   - Cork blocks offer stability and are eco-friendly.
   - For a softer option, high-density foam blocks are lightweight and comfortable.

4. **Straps:**
   - Look for cotton straps with a D-ring or quick-release buckle for easy adjustment.
   - An 8-10 foot strap offers versatility for different uses.

5. **Meditation Cushions:**
   - Choose a firm cushion filled with buckwheat hulls for stability and comfort.
   - Ensure the cover is removable and washable.

6. **Therapy Balls:**
   - Start with a set that includes different sizes (e.g., tennis ball, lacrosse ball, and softball sizes).
   - Look for balls with varying densities for different types of pressure work.

Tips for Choosing Comfortable Clothing for Somatic Practice

The right clothing can significantly enhance your somatic practice by allowing free movement and helping you focus on bodily sensations without distraction. Here are some tips to guide your choices:

1. **Prioritize Comfort:** Above all, choose clothes that feel good on your skin. Avoid

anything that pinches, binds, or restricts your movement in any way.

2. **Opt for Breathable Fabrics:** Natural fibers like cotton, bamboo, or moisture-wicking synthetic blends help keep you cool and comfortable during practice.

3. **Choose the Right Fit:**
   - Tops should be loose enough to allow full arm movement but not so baggy that they fall over your face in inverted positions.
   - Bottoms should allow for a full range of leg motion without slipping or bunching up.

4. **Consider Layering:** Wear layers that you can easily add or remove as your body temperature changes during practice.

5. **Avoid Distracting Elements:**
   - Steer clear of clothes with zippers, buttons, or scratchy tags that might dig into your skin during floor work.
   - Minimize loose or dangling elements like drawstrings or wide-leg pants that might get in your way.

6. **Think About Coverage:** Choose clothing that helps you feel secure and unselfconscious, allowing you to focus fully on your practice.

7. **Don't Forget Your Feet:** While many prefer bare feet for somatic work, have a pair of warm, comfortable socks nearby for cooler days or relaxation periods.

8. **Consider the Waistband:** Opt for bottoms with a comfortable, wide waistband that won't dig into your abdomen during bending or twisting movements.

9. **Test for Opacity:** If wearing leggings or fitted clothing, check that they remain opaque when stretched to avoid any wardrobe malfunctions during practice.

10. **Keep It Simple:** You don't need specialized or expensive "workout" clothes. Simple, comfortable items from your existing wardrobe often work perfectly well.

The ultimate goal is to wear clothing that allows you to forget about what you're wearing and focus entirely on your somatic experience. What works best can vary from person to person, so don't be afraid to experiment until you find what feels right for you.

Setting Realistic Goals

When most of us start something new, we put an insane amount of pressure on ourselves to excel from the get-go. We imagine dramatic transformations and quick results, setting ourselves up for disappointment if these lofty expectations aren't immediately met. However, when it comes to somatic exercise, this approach can be counterproductive and even discourage us from continuing our practice.

The beauty of somatic work lies in its subtlety and gradual nature, it simply just requires awareness, fostering a deeper connection with your body, and gently encouraging positive changes over time. With this in mind, it's crucial to set realistic, achievable goals that honor the true essence of somatic practice.

Here are some examples of realistic goals for your somatic exercise practice:

- **Consistency over intensity:** Aim to practice for 10-15 minutes daily rather than setting a goal for hour-long sessions three times a week.

- **Body awareness:** Set a goal to notice three new sensations in your body each week during your practice.

- **Stress reduction:** Aim to use a simple somatic technique, like conscious breathing or progressive muscle relaxation, once a day in response to stress.

- **Improved sleep:** Set a goal to incorporate a short somatic routine into your bedtime ritual three nights a week.

- **Pain management:** If you experience chronic pain, aim to reduce your pain levels by one point on a 1-10 scale over the course of a month through regular practice.

- **Mindfulness:** Strive to stay present and focused for one minute longer in each practice session.

- **Emotional regulation:** Set a goal to identify and name one emotion you feel in your body during each practice session.

- **Flexibility:** Aim to feel a slight increase in ease of movement in a particular area (like your shoulders or hips) over the course of a month.

- **Self-compassion:** Commit to responding to physical discomfort or limitations with kindness rather than frustration during your practice.

- **Integration:** Set a goal to apply one principle from your somatic practice (like mindful breathing or body scanning) to a daily activity each week.

Chapter 3: The Forms of Somatic Exercises

*To keep the body in good health is a duty... otherwise, we shall not be able to keep our mind strong and clear—*Buddha

Our bodies respond differently to different stimuli. Think about it—how you feel after a vigorous run is worlds apart from how you feel after a gentle stretch or a calming meditation. It's like our bodies speak multiple languages, each one unlocking a unique set of sensations and benefits.

Somatic exercises are no different. They come in various forms, each with its own 'dialect' that specifically communicates with your body. Some might make you feel grounded and centered like you're sinking roots deep into the earth. Others might leave you feeling light and free, as if a weight you didn't even know you were carrying has been lifted off your shoulders.

In this chapter, we'll explore these different forms of somatic exercises. Think of it as a tasting menu for your body and mind. We'll sample a bit of this and a bit of that, giving you a chance to discover which practices resonate with you the most. Maybe you'll find that slow, deliberate movements speak to your soul, or perhaps you'll discover that rhythmic, flowing exercises make your body sing.

The History of Somatic Exercise

The roots of somatic exercise stretch back to the early 20th century, intertwining with the development of modern dance, psychology, and a growing interest in mind-body connections. While the term "somatics" wasn't coined until the 1970s, its foundational principles were being explored decades earlier.

One of the pioneers in this field was F.M. Alexander, who developed the Alexander Technique in the 1890s. Alexander, an actor plagued by recurring voice loss, discovered that his posture and movement patterns were at the root of his problems. His work laid the groundwork for understanding how habitual patterns of tension affect our overall functioning.

In the 1920s and 30s, Moshe Feldenkrais, a physicist and judo practitioner, began developing his method after a debilitating knee injury. Feldenkrais combined his scientific knowledge with keen body awareness to create a system of gentle movements designed to improve physical and mental functioning.

Meanwhile, dancers like Mabel Elsworth Todd were exploring the connections between posture, movement, and emotion. Todd's work, which she called "Natural Posture," later evolved into Ideokinesis, an approach that uses imagery to change neuromuscular patterns.

The term "somatics" itself was coined by Thomas Hanna in the 1970s. Hanna, influenced by the work of Feldenkrais, developed Hanna Somatic Education, emphasizing the importance of internal physical perception and experience.

As these various methods developed and gained recognition, they began to influence fields beyond dance and theater, including psychology, physical therapy, and even traditional medicine. Today, somatic exercise encompasses a wide range of practices, all united by their focus on the internal experience of movement and the interconnection of mind and body.

How Somatics Work on the Nervous System

Somatic exercises work intimately with the nervous system, particularly the sensorimotor system, which governs our movement and our sense of our body in space. Here's a detailed look at how this interaction unfolds:

1. **Sensory-Motor Feedback Loop:** Somatic exercises enhance the feedback loop between our sensory neurons (which provide information about our body's position and movement) and our motor neurons (which control our muscles). By moving slowly and mindfully, we give our nervous system time to process this feedback more accurately, leading to improved body awareness and control.

2. **Neuroplasticity:** Regular practice of somatic exercises leverages neuroplasticity – the brain's ability to form new neural connections. As we repeatedly perform mindful movements, we create and strengthen neural pathways associated with these movements, potentially overriding habitual patterns of tension or misalignment.

3. **Interoception:** Somatic exercises heighten our interoceptive awareness – our ability to sense our internal bodily states. This increased awareness can help regulate the autonomic nervous system, potentially reducing stress and improving overall well-being.

4. **Proprioception:** These practices enhance proprioception – our sense of where our body is in space. Improved proprioception can lead to better balance, coordination, and overall movement efficiency.

5. **Muscular Re-education:** Many somatic techniques aim to release chronically tight muscles by first intentionally contracting them, then slowly releasing them. This process, known as pandiculation, helps reset the resting tone of muscles and can improve the nervous system's control over muscular tension.

6. **Autonomic Nervous System Regulation:** The slow, mindful nature of many somatic exercises can help shift the autonomic nervous system from sympathetic (fight-or-flight) dominance to parasympathetic (rest-and-digest) dominance. This shift can reduce stress, improve digestion, and promote overall relaxation.

7. **Cortical Remapping:** Focused attention on specific body parts during somatic exercises can lead to changes in how these parts are represented in the brain's somatosensory cortex. This "cortical remapping" can potentially help with pain management and improve motor control.

8. **Vagus Nerve Stimulation:** Some somatic practices, particularly those involving breath work or gentle movements of the neck and face, may stimulate the vagus nerve. This simulation can enhance parasympathetic activity, promoting a state of calm and improved stress resilience.

The Role of the Nervous System in Stress, Anxiety, and Tension

Your nervous system is the body's master control center. It's constantly monitoring your environment, both internal and external, and orchestrating responses to keep you safe and functioning optimally. When it comes to stress, anxiety, and tension, your nervous system plays a starring role in both creating and potentially alleviating these experiences. Let's break it down:

The Stress Response

When you encounter a stressor—whether it's a looming deadline, a near-miss in traffic, or even an exciting challenge—your nervous system springs into action:

1. **The Amygdala Sounds the Alarm:** This almond-shaped structure in your brain is like your emotional smoke detector. It detects potential threats and signals the hypothalamus to activate the stress response.

2. **The HPA Axis Kicks In:** The hypothalamus activates the hypothalamic-pituitary-adrenal (HPA) axis, triggering a hormonal cascade. Cortisol, the primary stress

hormone, is released, preparing your body for action.

3. **The Sympathetic Nervous System Takes the Wheel:** Part of your autonomic nervous system, the sympathetic branch initiates the "fight-or-flight" response. It increases heart rate, boosts blood flow to muscles, and sharpens focus.

4. **Physical Tension Builds:** Muscles tense up as part of this preparatory response, ready for action if needed.

Chronic Tension: The Body's Stress Memory

Ongoing stress and anxiety can lead to chronic muscle tension, which itself becomes a source of stress:

1. **Muscle Memory:** Repeated tensing of muscles in response to stress can become habitual, with the nervous system maintaining this tension even when the stressor is gone.

2. **Pain-Tension Cycle:** Chronic tension can lead to pain, which signals the nervous system to create more tension as a protective measure, creating a self-perpetuating cycle.

3. **Sensorimotor Amnesia:** A term coined by Thomas Hanna, this refers to the loss of awareness of chronically tense muscles, making it difficult to consciously relax them.

The Potential for Relief

Understanding the nervous system's role in stress, anxiety, and tension is empowering because it points to potential solutions:

1. **Vagus Nerve Stimulation:** Activating the vagus nerve, a key part of the parasympathetic nervous system, can help shift the body out of stress mode and into a state of relaxation.

2. **Interoceptive Awareness:** Improving our ability to sense internal bodily states can help us recognize and respond to stress signals earlier.

3. **Neuroplasticity:** The brain's ability to form new neural connections means we can potentially rewire our stress responses through practices like mindfulness and somatic exercises.

4. **HRV Training:** Heart Rate Variability training can help balance the autonomic nervous system, improving our ability to cope with stress.

5. **Somatic Exercises:** These can help relieve chronic muscle tension, improve body awareness, and promote overall nervous system regulation.

Pioneers of Somatic Exercise: Hanna, Feldenkrais, and Alexander

The world of somatic exercise owes much to three visionary thinkers: Thomas Hanna, Moshe Feldenkrais, and F.M. Alexander. Each of these pioneers brought unique insights to the field, shaping the way we understand the connection between mind and body.

Thomas Hanna: The Name of Somatics

Thomas Hanna (1928-1990) didn't just contribute to the field of somatics—he gave it its name. He believed that many of our physical limitations and pains weren't due to aging or injury but to learned movement patterns and posture. He called this "sensory-motor amnesia"—essentially, our bodies forgetting how to move efficiently.

He developed a method called "Somatic Education," which uses slow, gentle movements and focused attention to help people regain awareness and control of their bodies. His approach focuses on resetting your body's operating system, by helping you unlearn harmful habits and rediscover more natural, comfortable ways of moving.

Though his contributions to the field of somatics have been groundbreaking, like many pioneering ideas, they've sometimes been misunderstood or oversimplified. Here are the common myths surrounding Hanna's work and then clarify the realities.

Myth 1: Hanna Somatics Can Cure All Physical Ailments

Some enthusiasts claim that Hanna Somatics is a panacea for all physical problems.

Reality: While Hanna Somatics can be incredibly effective for many issues, particularly those related to muscular tension and movement patterns, it's not a cure-all. Hanna himself never claimed it could solve every physical problem, it's merely a tool for addressing certain types of chronic pain and movement limitations, but it works best as part of a comprehensive approach to health and wellness.

Myth 2: Hanna's Work is Just Another Form of Stretching

Some people mistakenly equate Hanna Somatics with simple stretching exercises.

Reality: Hanna Somatics is fundamentally different from traditional stretching. It focuses on retraining the nervous system's control of muscles through a process called pandiculation—a combination of gentle contraction and slow, mindful release. This approach aims to reset the resting tone of muscles and improve the brain's ability to sense and control them, going far beyond what stretching alone can achieve.

Myth 3: Somatic Exercises Are Only for the Elderly or Those in Pain

There's a misconception that Hanna's methods are only beneficial for older adults or those suffering from chronic pain.

Reality: While Hanna's work can indeed be transformative for these groups, it's valuable for people of all ages and fitness levels. Athletes use it to enhance performance and prevent injuries. Office workers find it helpful for countering the effects of prolonged sitting. Even children can benefit from improved body awareness and movement efficiency.

Myth 4: Hanna Claimed to Have Invented Somatics

Some believe that Hanna presented himself as the sole creator of the field of somatics.

Reality: Hanna coined the term "somatics" and significantly developed the field, but he always acknowledged his influences, including the work of Feldenkrais and others. He saw himself as part of a broader movement exploring the mind-body connection, not as its sole originator.

Myth 5: Hanna Somatics Requires No Effort

There's a misconception that because the movements are gentle, they don't require effort or commitment.

Reality: While Hanna Somatics doesn't involve strenuous physical exertion, it does require focused mental effort and consistent practice. The subtle nature of the work demands attention and patience. Real change comes from regular practice and the gradual reprogramming of neuromuscular patterns.

Myth 6: Hanna's Ideas Aren't Scientifically Supported

Some critics argue that Hanna's work lacks scientific backing.

Reality: While it's true that when Hanna first developed his ideas, there wasn't a wealth of scientific research to support them, this has changed. Many of Hanna's core concepts, such as the plasticity of the nervous system and the role of movement in pain management, are now supported by neuroscientific research. However, as with many mind-body approaches, more research is always welcome to further understand and validate the mechanisms at play.

Thomas Hanna's work was without a doubt, truly revolutionary, but it's important to approach his work, like any method, with a balanced perspective. It's a tool for improving body awareness, reducing chronic pain, and enhancing movement quality, but it's most effective when integrated with other health practices and viewed as part of a holistic approach to well-being.

Moshe Feldenkrais: The Physicist of Movement

Moshe Feldenkrais (1904-1984) was a true Renaissance man: a physicist, engineer, martial artist, and movement pioneer. After suffering a debilitating knee injury, he applied his analytical mind to the problem of human movement and healing. He developed two complementary methods: Functional Integration (hands-on, one-on-one sessions) and Awareness Through Movement (verbally guided group classes). Both aim to improve movement and function by increasing body awareness and exploring new movement patterns.

Feldenkrais's approach is all about learning—not exercising or correcting. He believed that if you give the nervous system better information, it will naturally choose more efficient, comfortable ways of moving—like upgrading your body's software by expanding its movement vocabulary.

F.M. Alexander: The Posture Pioneer

Frederick Matthias Alexander (1869-1955) was an Australian actor who developed vocal problems that threatened his career. Alexander discovered that his vocal issues were linked to his overall posture and the way he held tension in his body. He developed a technique to consciously improve posture and reduce unnecessary tension, particularly in the head, neck, and back.

The Alexander Technique, as it came to be known, is about becoming aware of habitual ways of holding and moving your body that may be causing pain or limiting your function. It's like learning to read the user manual for your own body, understanding how your thoughts and intentions translate into physical actions.

The Common Thread

While Hanna, Feldenkrais, and Alexander developed distinct methods, they share common principles:

1. **Mindfulness:** All three emphasize the importance of paying attention to what

you're doing with your body.

2. **Neuroplasticity:** They recognized, before it was scientifically proven, that the brain can change and that movement patterns can be relearned.

3. **Holistic Approach:** Each saw the body and mind as an interconnected whole, not separate entities.

4. **Gentle Exploration:** Rather than forceful exercise, they advocated for gentle, mindful movement to create change.

5. **Empowerment:** All three methods aim to give people tools to help themselves rather than relying solely on a practitioner.

Some questions have been stirring lately: How much joy can a nervous system hold? How much pleasure can it contain? How much kindness can it embrace? How much slowness can it savor?

I am learning that we can gradually expand our capacity for stillness, slowness, for softness because the nervous system is a living, breathing entity—one that can expand, soften, and grow. With each breath, each mindful movement, the boundaries of bodily experience stretch ever so slightly, gently coaxing the body to open up, to let in more of life's richness.

Chapter 4: Managing Anxiety with Somatic Exercise

In the rhythm of movement, anxiety loses its grip; each breath, each step, a return to calm.—Tara Zen

I read somewhere that anxiety is basically living in the future. It's your mind time-traveling to all the "what ifs" and worst-case scenarios. All of this made me think that I was broken somehow. Why couldn't I just "stop worrying" like everyone told me to? It wasn't until I discovered somatic exercises that I realized my body wasn't the enemy – it was trying to be my ally all along.

The turning point came with one simple practice. Whenever I feel uncertain or not at ease, I place my hand on my chest. It's such a small gesture, but it's like hitting a reset button on my nervous system. As I feel my own heartbeat beneath my palm, I remind myself: "Uncertainty is where possibility lives. Uncertainty is where freedom lives."

At first, it felt strange. How could acknowledging uncertainty bring comfort? But as I practiced this, something shifted. That hand on my chest became a bridge between my racing thoughts and my physical sensations. It brought me back to the present moment, where anxiety couldn't survive.

I began to notice how anxiety lived in my body—the tight chest, the shallow breathing, the clenched jaw. But instead of these sensations spiraling me into panic, they became signals to pause, breathe, and remember that uncertainty isn't my enemy.

This simple somatic practice didn't make my anxiety disappear overnight. There are still moments when worry creeps in. But now, instead of getting swept away by it, I have a tool to ground myself. I've learned to befriend my body and listen to its wisdom.

Understanding Anxiety and Its Triggers

Grocery stores used to be a sensitive point for me—yes, grocery stores. The fluorescent lights, the endless aisles, the decision fatigue of choosing between 15 different types of peanut butter—it all conspired to send my anxiety skyrocketing. My heart would race, my palms would sweat, and more than once, I abandoned a full cart in the middle of the store, fleeing to the safety of my car. It wasn't rational, and I knew it, but anxiety rarely cares about rationality.

What I didn't realize then was that my body was trying to tell me something. Those physical symptoms—the racing heart, the sweaty palms, the overwhelming urge to escape—were my nervous system's way of saying, "Hey, something doesn't feel safe here." It wasn't about the groceries at all. The store had become a trigger, a place where my body remembered past stress and anticipated future discomfort.

Anxiety is an interplay of physiological and psychological factors. Physiologically, it's rooted in our body's stress response system. When we perceive a threat, real or imagined, our amygdala—the brain's alarm system—sends out distress signals that trigger a cascade of hormones, including adrenaline and cortisol, preparing our body for fight, flight, or freeze. Our heart rate increases, breathing quickens, and muscles tense. It's an ancient survival mechanism, incredibly useful when facing actual danger, but often overwhelming in modern life, where threats are more often psychological than physical.

Psychologically, it often manifests as persistent worry, intrusive thoughts, and a sense of impending doom. It distorts our perception and makes us hyper-focus on potential threats and worst-case scenarios. This cognitive aspect of anxiety can create a feedback loop with the physiological symptoms, each reinforcing the other. Our racing thoughts fuel our racing hearts, which in turn convinces our minds that there must be something to worry about. Breaking this cycle requires addressing both the mind and the body, which is where somatic exercises can be particularly effective.

Common anxiety triggers can vary widely from person to person, but some frequently reported ones include:

1. **Social situations:** For many, interactions with others, especially in large groups or with strangers, can trigger anxiety.
2. **Performance pressure:** Work presentations, exams, or any situation where you feel you're being evaluated can be anxiety-inducing.
3. **Health concerns:** Worrying about personal health or the health of loved ones is a common trigger, especially in times of global health crises.

4. **Financial stress:** Money worries, job insecurity, or significant financial decisions can all trigger anxiety.

5. **Major life changes:** Even positive changes like moving, starting a new job, or getting married can trigger anxiety due to the uncertainty involved.

6. **Conflict:** Interpersonal conflicts or the anticipation of difficult conversations can be significant triggers.

7. **Specific phobias:** Particular objects or situations, like heights, enclosed spaces, or certain animals, can trigger intense anxiety in some people.

8. **Trauma reminders:** For those who've experienced trauma, situations, sounds, or sensations reminiscent of the traumatic event can trigger anxiety.

9. **Decision-making:** For some, having to make decisions, especially important ones, can trigger anxiety.

10. **Lack of control:** Situations where we feel we have little or no control can be particularly anxiety-inducing.

Somatic Movement for Anxiety Relief

Before you start working through the exercises, remember that you can scan the QR code in the beginning of the book for a more detailed, more visual interpretation of the exercises. May your journey be restorative, healing, soothing, and incredibly rewarding!

Here is the QR code again as a quick reminder.

The body loves movement. It craves it, thrives on it, and uses it as a language to communicate with us. When we engage in mindful, intentional movements, we create a dialogue with our body; we give it a chance to express itself, release pent-up tension, and find its way back to balance. Somatic movements for anxiety relief invite you to tune in, listen attentively, and allow your body to guide you toward a state of calm. In this section, we'll explore how simple movements can become powerful tools for managing anxiety, helping you not just cope with stress but move through it with grace and resilience.

Cat-Cow Pose (Marjaryasana-Bitilasana)

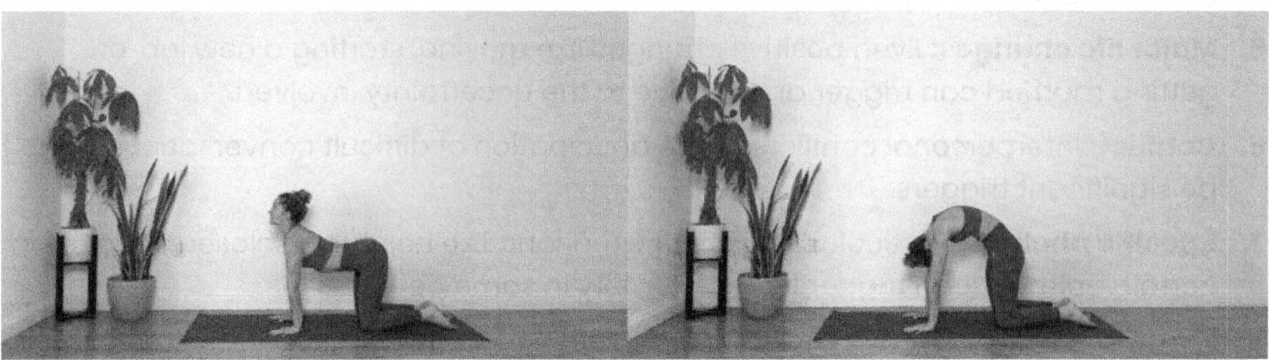

Cat-Cow is a gentle, accessible yoga pose that warms up the spine and brings flexibility to the neck, shoulders, and torso. It's excellent for relieving tension and calming the mind through rhythmic movement and breath.

1. Start on your hands and knees in a "tabletop" position. Your wrists should be under your shoulders, and your knees under your hips.

2. Begin with Cat Pose: As you exhale, round your spine toward the ceiling, tucking your chin to your chest and drawing your navel toward your spine.

3. Move into Cow Pose: As you inhale, arch your back, lifting your chest and tailbone toward the ceiling. Let your belly relax toward the floor and lift your gaze.

4. Continue this fluid movement, coordinating your breath with each motion. Exhale for Cat, inhale for Cow.

5. Repeat for 5-10 cycles, moving slowly and mindfully.

Dynamic Child's Pose (Balasana) with Arm Reaches

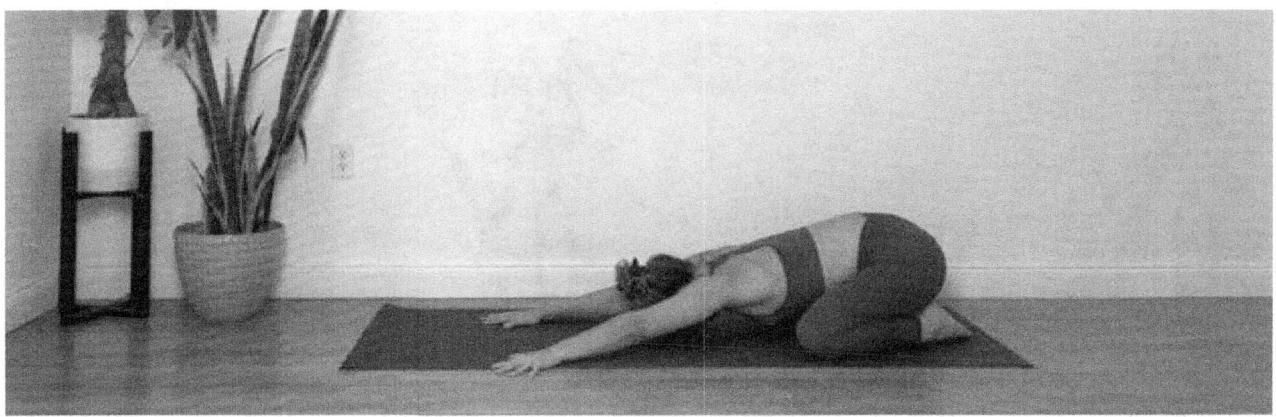

This is a variation of the traditional Child's Pose that incorporates arm movements. It helps release tension in the back, shoulders, and hips while promoting a sense of grounding and safety.

1. Start in a kneeling position, then sit back on your heels.

2. Fold forward, lowering your chest toward your thighs and extending your arms out in front of you.

3. Take a few deep breaths here, feeling the stretch in your back.

4. As you inhale, sweep your right arm up and to the right, creating a half-circle motion.

5. Exhale as you bring the arm back down to the starting position.

6. Repeat with the left arm.

7. Continue alternating arms for 5-10 cycles on each side, moving slowly and breathing deeply.

Spinal Rolls (Seated or Standing)

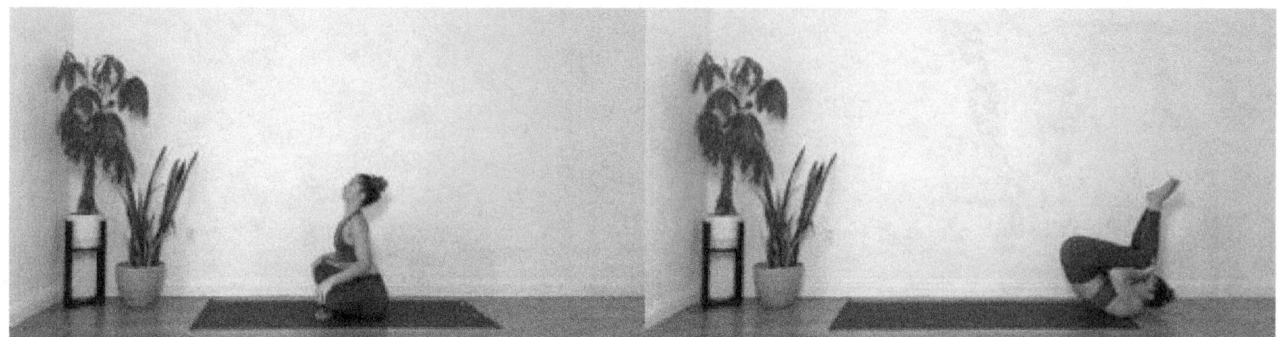

Spinal rolls are a gentle way to release tension throughout the entire spine. They can be done seated or standing and help improve posture, increase spinal mobility, and promote relaxation.

1. Sit on the floor with your legs crossed comfortably.

2. Place your hands on your knees or thighs.

3. As you inhale, lift your chest, arch your back slightly, and look up toward the ceiling.

4. As you exhale, round your spine, tucking your chin to your chest and drawing your navel toward your spine.

5. Continue this rolling motion, moving slowly and mindfully with your breath.

6. Repeat for 5–10 cycles.

Steps for Standing Spinal Rolls

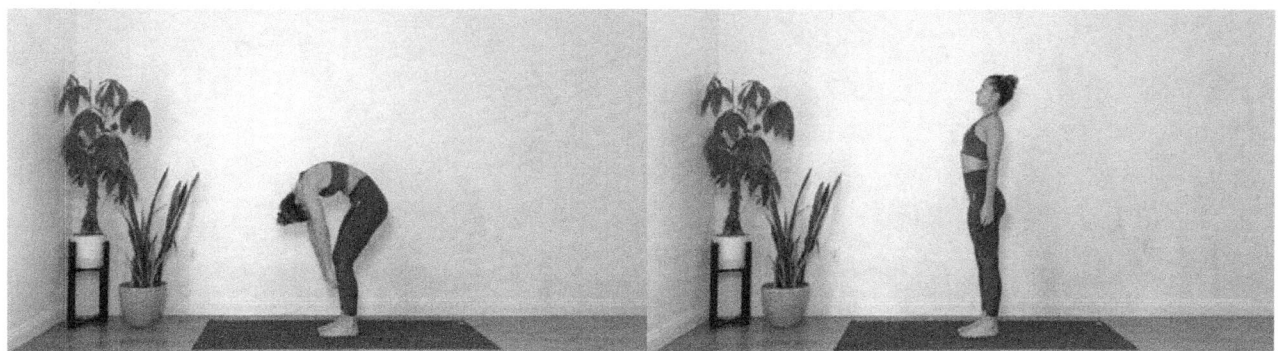

1. Stand with your feet hip-width apart, knees slightly bent.

2. As you inhale, roll your shoulders back, lift your chest, and look up toward the ceiling.

3. As you exhale, round your spine, tucking your chin to your chest and reaching your arms forward.

4. Continue this rolling motion, moving slowly and mindfully with your breath.

5. Let your arms hang loosely, moving naturally with the motion of your spine.

6. Repeat for 5-10 cycles.

Pelvic Tilts

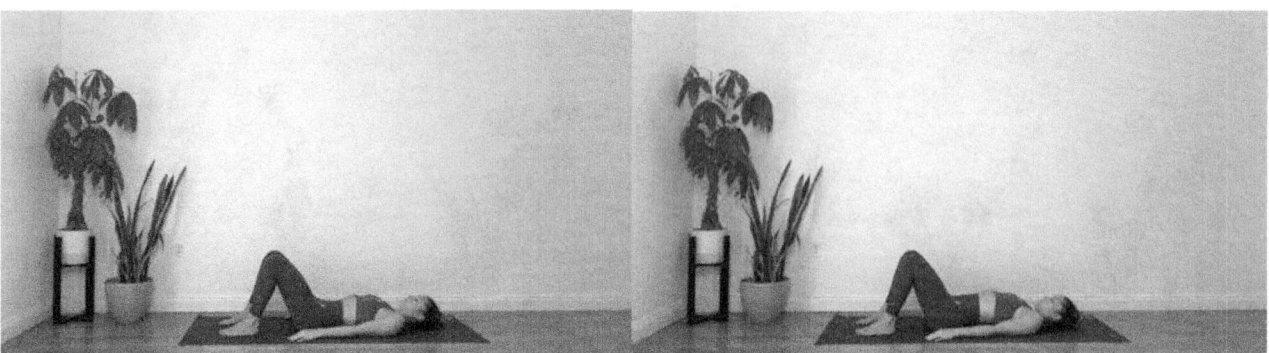

Pelvic tilts are a gentle exercise that helps release tension in the lower back and abdominal muscles. This movement increases awareness of the pelvis and its relationship to the spine, promoting better posture and reducing anxiety-related tension.

1. Lie on your back with your knees bent and feet flat on the floor, hip-width apart.

2. Place your arms by your sides, palms down.

3. Inhale and allow your belly to rise.

4. As you exhale, gently tilt your pelvis upward, pressing your lower back into the floor. Feel your abdominal muscles engage.

5. Inhale and return to the neutral position, allowing your lower back to lift slightly off the floor.

6. Repeat this movement slowly for 10-15 cycles, coordinating with your breath.

Gentle Neck Rolls

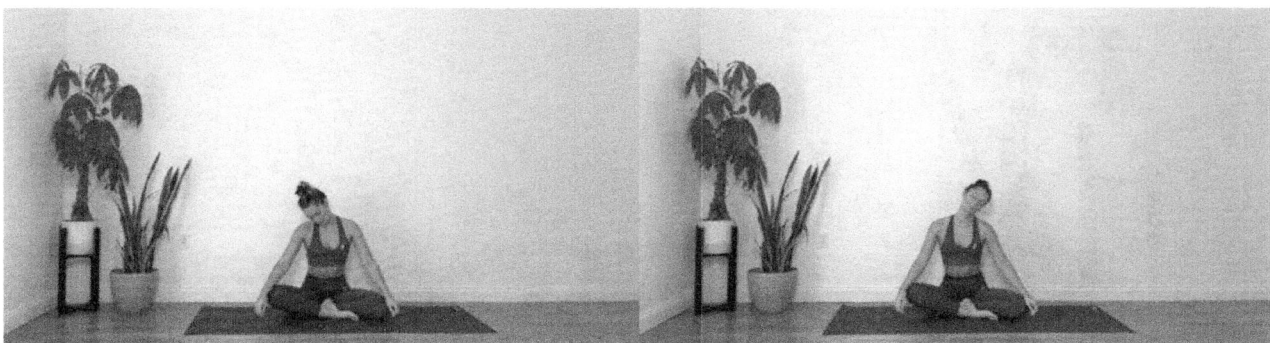

Neck rolls help release tension in the neck and shoulders, areas where many people hold stress and anxiety. This exercise promotes relaxation and increases the range of motion in the cervical spine.

1. Sit comfortably with your spine straight, either on the floor or in a chair.

2. Allow your chin to drop toward your chest, feeling a stretch in the back of your neck.

3. Slowly roll your head to the right, bringing your right ear toward your right shoulder.

4. Continue the roll, bringing your head back so you're looking at the ceiling.

5. Complete the circle by rolling to the left, bringing your left ear toward your left shoulder, and then back to the starting position.

6. Repeat this circle 3-5 times, then reverse the direction for another 3-5 circles.

7. Move slowly and gently, stopping if you feel any pain or dizziness.

Constructive Rest Position

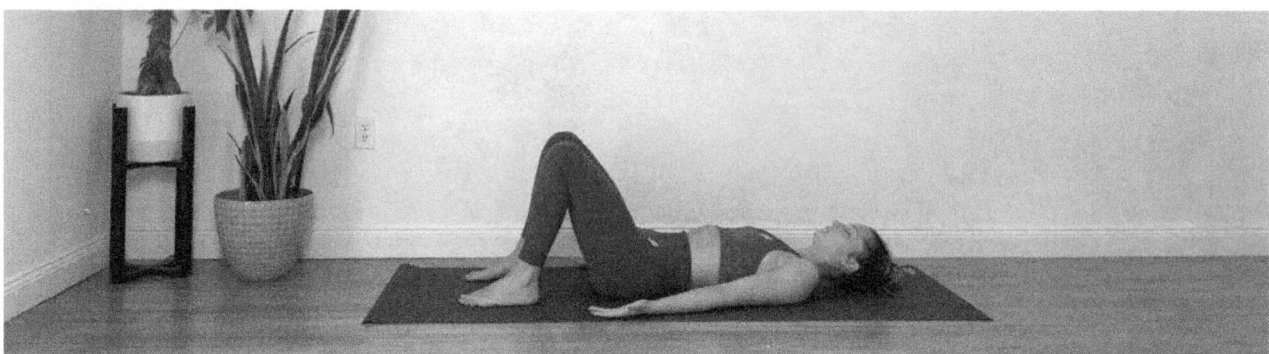

The Constructive Rest Position is a passive pose that allows the body to release tension and realign naturally. It's excellent for calming the nervous system and reducing anxiety.

1. Lie on your back on a flat surface.

2. Bend your knees and place your feet flat on the floor, about hip-width apart.

3. Let your arms rest by your sides, palms facing up.

4. Close your eyes and focus on your breath, allowing your body to settle into the floor.

5. Notice any areas of tension and consciously allow them to relax.

6. Remain in this position for 5-15 minutes, or longer if comfortable.

Arch and Flatten

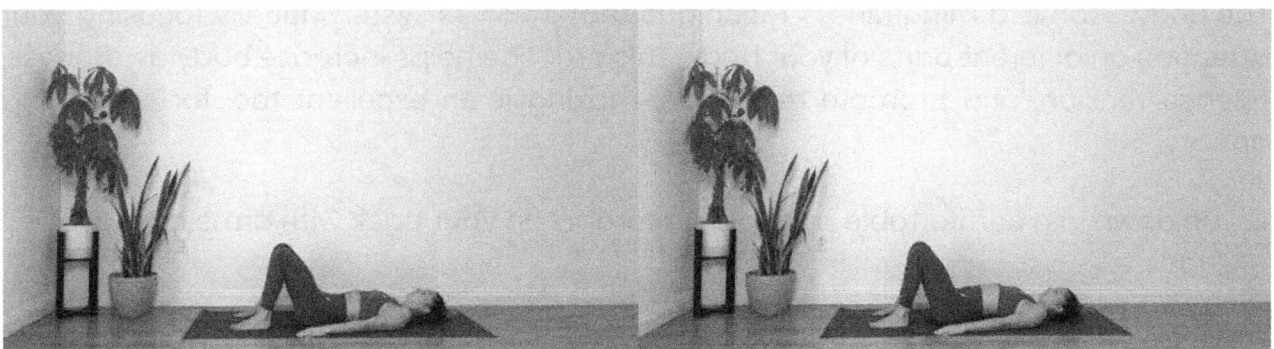

This exercise increases awareness of the lumbar spine and strengthens the core muscles. It can help release lower back tension and promote a sense of grounding, which is beneficial for anxiety relief.

1. Lie on your back with your knees bent and feet flat on the floor, hip-width apart.

2. Place your arms by your sides, palms down.

3. Inhale and gently arch your lower back, creating a small space between your lower back and the floor.

4. Exhale and flatten your lower back against the floor, engaging your abdominal muscles.

5. Inhale to arch, exhale to flatten.

6. Repeat this movement slowly for 10-15 cycles, coordinating with your breath.

7. Focus on the sensation of your spine moving and the engagement of your core muscles.

Body Scan

The Body Scan is a mindfulness technique that involves systematically focusing your attention on different parts of your body. This practice helps increase body awareness, release tension, and promote relaxation, making it an excellent tool for managing anxiety.

1. Lie down in a comfortable position, preferably on your back with arms at your sides.

2. Close your eyes and take a few deep breaths to center yourself.

3. Begin by focusing your attention on your toes. Notice any sensations without trying to change them.

4. Slowly move your attention up through your feet, ankles, calves, knees, thighs, and so on, all the way up to the top of your head.

5. At each body part, pause for a few moments. Notice any sensations, tension, or emotions stored there.

6. If you notice areas of tension, imagine breathing into that area and allowing it to soften and release.

7. Continue this process until you've scanned your entire body.

8. Finish by taking a few deep breaths and slowly opening your eyes.

This exercise can take anywhere from 5 to 30 minutes, depending on how detailed you make your scan.

Progressive Muscle Relaxation

PMR is a technique that involves tensing and then relaxing different muscle groups in the body. This practice helps you distinguish between tension and relaxation, allowing you to release physical stress more effectively. This exercise typically takes about 15-20 minutes to complete.

1. Find a comfortable position, either sitting or lying down.

2. Start with your feet. Curl your toes and tense the muscles in your feet for 5 seconds.

3. Release the tension all at once, and notice the feeling of relaxation for 10-15 seconds.

4. Move up to your calves. Tense these muscles for 5 seconds, then release.

5. Continue this process, moving up through your body: thighs, buttocks, abdomen, chest, arms, hands, shoulders, neck, and face.

6. For each muscle group, tense for 5 seconds and relax for 10-15 seconds.

7. Pay attention to the differences between tension and relaxation in each area.

8. After you've completed the whole body, take a few deep breaths and notice how your body feels.

Grounding Techniques

Grounding techniques are practices that help you connect with the present moment and your physical surroundings. They're particularly useful for managing anxiety, panic attacks, or dissociation.

5-4-3-2-1 Technique:

1. Find a comfortable seated position.

2. Take a few deep breaths to center yourself.

3. Look around you and name (out loud or in your head):

   - 5 things you can see
   - 4 things you can touch
   - 3 things you can hear
   - 2 things you can smell
   - 1 thing you can taste

4. Take your time with each sense, really focusing on the details of each thing you notice.

Physical Grounding:

1. Stand barefoot on the ground, preferably outdoors on grass or soil.

2. Focus on the sensation of your feet connecting with the ground.

3. Imagine roots growing from the soles of your feet, anchoring you to the earth.

4. Take slow, deep breaths, visualizing energy flowing up from the earth through your feet and into your body.

5. Continue for 5-10 minutes, or until you feel more centered and calm.

Somatic Twists

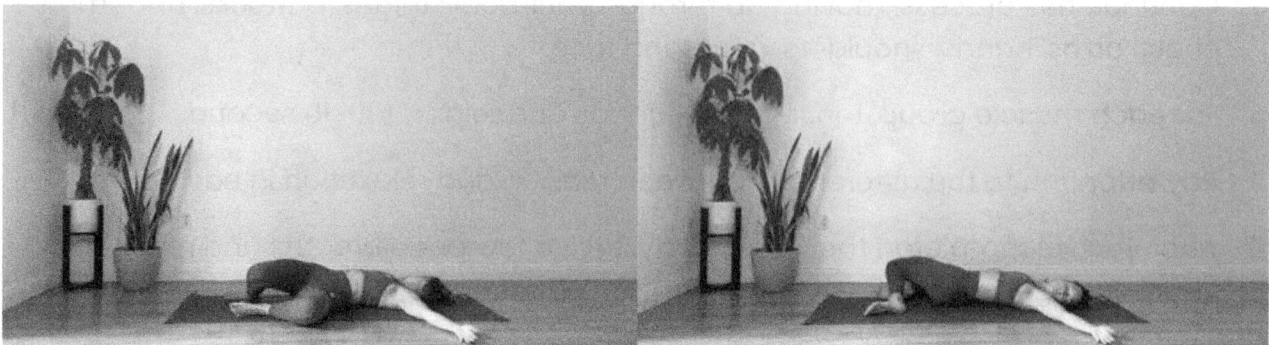

Somatic twists are gentle spinal rotations that help release tension in the back, improve spinal mobility, and promote relaxation. They can be particularly effective for relieving anxiety-related tension held in the back and core.

1. Lie on your back with your knees bent and feet flat on the floor, hip-width apart.

2. Extend your arms out to the sides, forming a T-shape with your body.

3. Keeping your shoulders flat on the floor, gently let both knees fall to the right side.

4. Turn your head to the left, creating a gentle twist through your spine.

5. Hold for 5-10 deep breaths, feeling the stretch and release.

6. Slowly bring your knees and head back to the center.

7. Repeat on the other side, letting your knees fall to the left and turning your head to the right.

8. Perform 3-5 repetitions on each side, moving slowly and mindfully.

Tabletop Arm and Leg Extensions

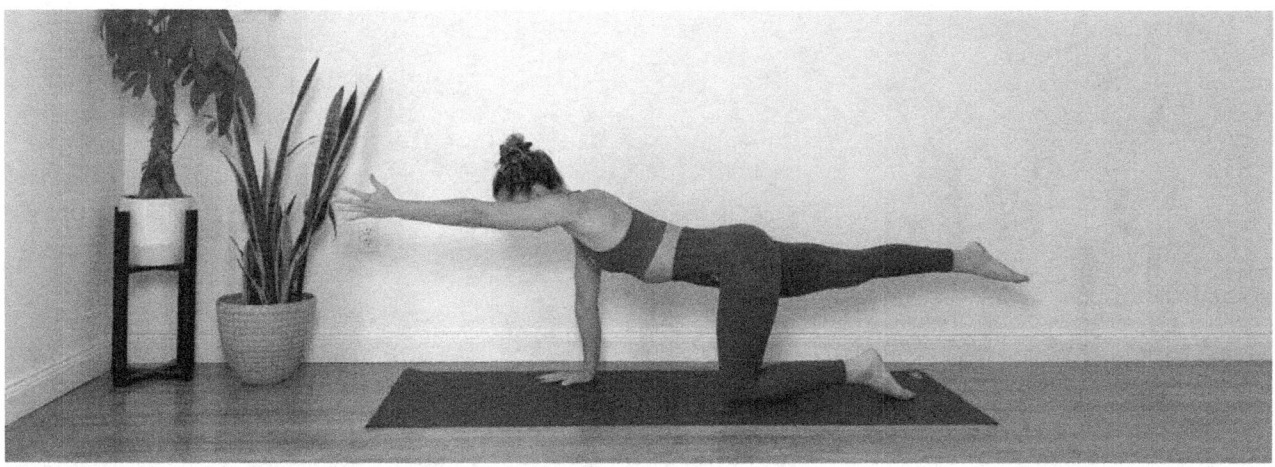

This exercise, also known as "Bird Dog," improves balance, strengthens the core, and promotes mind-body connection. It can help reduce anxiety by encouraging focus and controlled movement.

Steps:

1. Start on your hands and knees in a tabletop position. Your wrists should be under your shoulders, and your knees under your hips.

2. Extend your right arm forward while simultaneously extending your left leg back.

3. Hold this position for 3-5 breaths, focusing on maintaining balance and keeping your core engaged.

4. Slowly return to the starting position.

5. Repeat with the left arm and right leg.

6. Perform 5-10 repetitions on each side, moving slowly and with control.

Sphinx Pose

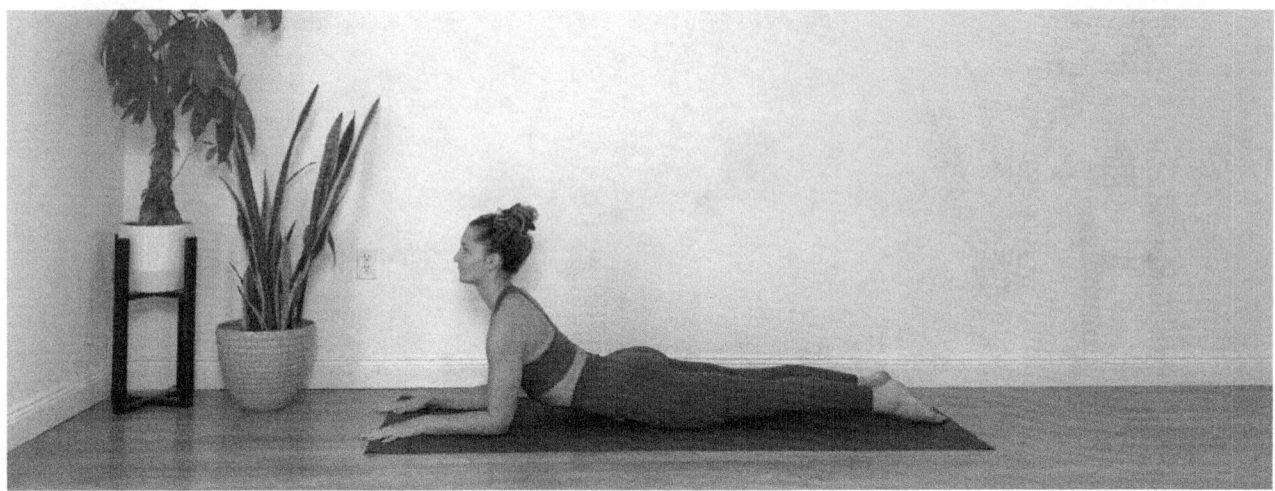

Sphinx pose is a gentle backbend that opens the chest, strengthens the spine, and can help alleviate anxiety by encouraging deep breathing and releasing tension in the upper body.

Steps:

1. Lie on your stomach with your legs extended behind you.

2. Place your elbows under your shoulders, and forearms on the floor.

3. Lift your upper body, keeping your hips and legs on the floor.

4. Draw your shoulder blades down your back and lift your chest.

5. Keep your gaze forward or slightly downward to maintain a long, neutral neck.

6. Hold this position for 5-10 deep breaths, focusing on the expansion of your chest with each inhale.

7. To release, slowly lower your upper body back to the floor.

8. Rest for a few breaths before repeating 2-3 times if comfortable.

Side-Lying Leg Lifts

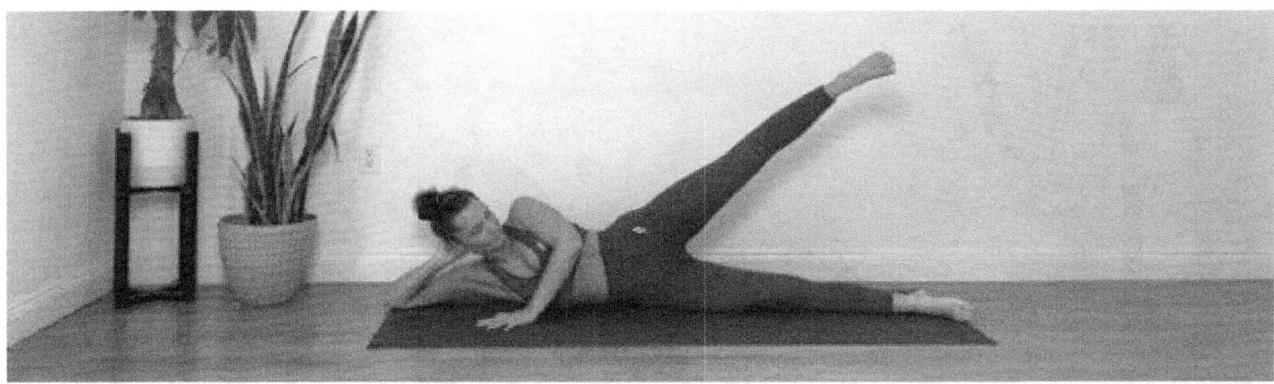

This exercise strengthens the hips and outer thighs while promoting body awareness. It can help ground you in your body, which is beneficial for managing anxiety.

Steps:

1. Lie on your right side with your legs stacked and knees slightly bent.

2. Support your head with your right hand or rest it on your arm.

3. Place your left hand on the floor in front of you for balance.

4. Keeping your hips stacked, slowly lift your left leg about 45 degrees.

5. Hold for a moment at the top, then slowly lower.

6. Repeat for 10–15 repetitions.

7. Turn onto your left side and repeat with your right leg.

8. Focus on the sensation in your hips and legs, using the movement to anchor your attention.

Somatic Shoulder Shrugs

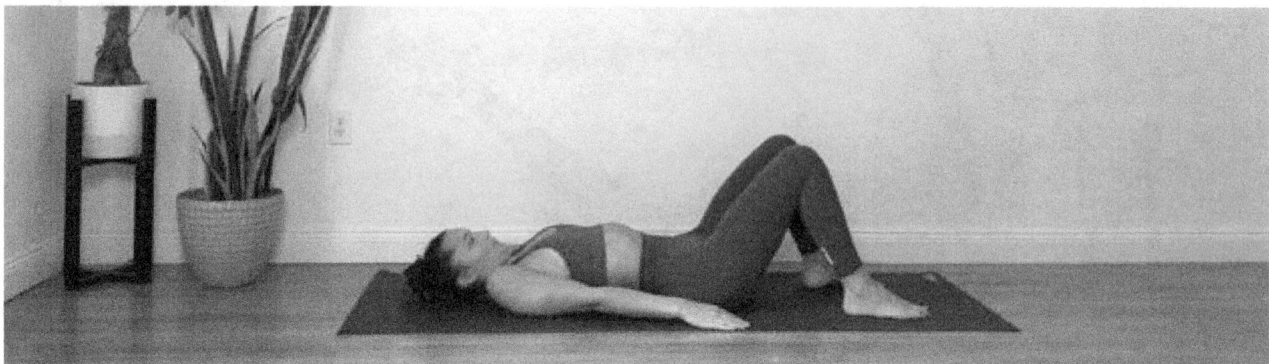

This exercise helps release tension in the shoulders and neck, areas where many people hold stress and anxiety. It promotes relaxation and increases body awareness.

1. Lie on your back with your knees bent and feet flat on the floor.

2. Let your arms rest comfortably by your sides, palms facing down.

3. As you inhale, slowly shrug your shoulders up towards your ears.

4. As you exhale, slowly release your shoulders back down, letting them melt into the floor.

5. Pay close attention to the sensation of tension as you lift and the release as you lower.

6. Repeat this movement for 10-15 breaths, coordinating with your breath.

7. After the final repetition, let your shoulders rest heavily on the floor and notice the difference in sensation.

Breathing Techniques for Anxiety Management

There is power in breath, in counting steadily and rhythmically while you inhale and exhale. It's something simple; something that we do thousands of times a day without thinking, but when harnessed intentionally, it becomes a potent tool for managing anxiety. Your breath is an anchor, always there, always accessible, ready to ground you in stress or panic.

When anxiety strikes, our breathing often becomes shallow and rapid, feeding into the cycle of tension and worry, but by consciously controlling our breath, we can send a powerful message to our nervous system. Slow, deep breaths tell our body that we're safe, that there's no need for the fight-or-flight response. It gives you a direct line to your body's relaxation response, a way to manually override the anxiety alarm that's been accidentally triggered.

The beauty of breathing techniques lies in their simplicity and accessibility. You don't need any special equipment or a quiet room. Whether you're in a crowded subway, a high-stakes meeting, or lying awake at night, your breath is always with you, a silent ally in your battle against anxiety. In this section, we'll explore various breathing techniques that can help you tap into this innate superpower, giving you practical tools to find calm amidst the chaos of anxiety.

Box Breathing (Square Breathing)

Box breathing is a simple yet effective technique that can help calm your nervous system and improve focus.

1. Sit comfortably with your back straight.

2. Exhale slowly, getting all the air out of your lungs.

3. Inhale slowly through your nose for a count of 4.

4. Hold your breath for a count of 4.

5. Exhale slowly through your mouth for a count of 4.

6. Hold your breath for a count of 4.

7. Repeat this cycle for 4-5 minutes or until you feel calmer.

4-7-8 Breathing

This exercise, developed by Dr. Andrew Weil, acts as a natural tranquilizer for the nervous system.

1. Sit with your back straight.

2. Place the tip of your tongue against the ridge behind your upper front teeth.

3. Exhale completely through your mouth, making a whoosh sound.

4. Close your mouth and inhale quietly through your nose for a count of 4.

5. Hold your breath for a count of 7.

6. Exhale completely through your mouth, making a whoosh sound, for a count of 8.

7. Repeat this cycle for a total of 4 breaths.

Alternate Nostril Breathing (Nadi Shodhana)

This technique from yoga helps balance the left and right hemispheres of the brain and can be particularly calming.

1. Sit comfortably with your back straight.

2. Use your right thumb to close your right nostril.

3. Inhale deeply through your left nostril.

4. At the peak of inhalation, close off the left nostril with your ring finger, release the right nostril, and exhale through the right side.

5. Inhale through the right nostril.

6. At the peak of inhalation, close off the right nostril and exhale through the left.

7. This completes one cycle. Repeat for 5-10 cycles.

Deep Belly Breathing (Diaphragmatic Breathing)

This deep breathing technique helps activate the body's relaxation response by engaging the diaphragm fully.

1. Lie on your back with your knees bent and feet flat on the floor.

2. Place one hand on your upper chest and the other just below your rib cage.

3. Breathe in slowly through your nose, feeling your stomach rise against your lower hand. Your upper hand should remain as still as possible.

4. Tighten your stomach muscles and let them fall inward as you exhale through pursed lips. The hand on your upper chest should remain still.

5. Repeat for 5-10 minutes.

Remember, the key to any and all exercise is practice. You'll feel a bit awkward at first, but with regular use, they'll become more natural and effective. Start by practicing when you're calm, so you can easily access these techniques when anxiety strikes. Always breathe at a pace that feels comfortable for you, and never force your breath in a way that causes discomfort.

Chapter 5: Stress Relief Through Somatic Exercise

Move your body to free your mind; in physical release lies mental peace.—Tara Zen

They say that at rest, the human body carries just about enough energy to power up a small city. Now I am no scientist or anything like that, I am a writer, but I have concluded, from this scientific evidence, that it's all of us walking around like tiny power plants, buzzing with energy and you know what else? I am convinced from this scientific evidence that when we're all rested, it's all of us who are keeping the skies so brightly lit up at night.

Sometimes, all that energy gets unruly; we become walking, talking bundles of electricity, but instead of lighting up the sky, we're shorting out our own circuits. Those days when everything feels like it's just too much, when the simplest task feels like moving mountains, and your brain is buzzing louder than a swarm of angry bees, that's your inner power plant going haywire. I'm not saying we need to shut down our personal power stations. Far from it. We need a way to channel all that energy, to smooth out the spikes and dips. You don't need to add more to your already full plate. Instead, you listen to your body, feeling where that energy is stuck or overflowing, and gently guiding it back into balance. In this chapter, we're going to explore how you can use these gentle, mindful movements to transform stress from a chaotic lightning storm into a steady, warm glow.

External and Internal Stressors

We're all walking around with two different stress radars: one scanning the outside world, and another keeping tabs on what's going on inside us. Let's break these down into external and internal stressors.

External Stressors

External stressors come from things that are outside ourselves; they'll often feel like they're beyond our control. These are the things in our environment or circumstances that put pressure on us and trigger our stress response.

Common external stressors include:

- Work-related pressures (deadlines, difficult bosses, heavy workloads)
- Financial problems (debt, unexpected expenses, job loss)
- Relationship issues (conflicts with partners, family members, or friends)
- Major life changes (moving, getting married, having a baby)
- Environmental factors (noise pollution, crowded spaces, extreme weather)
- News and world events (political unrest, natural disasters, pandemics)
- Time pressures and busy schedules
- Traffic and commuting issues
- Social obligations and expectations
- Academic pressures (exams, assignments, college applications)

These external stressors are often the ones we vent about to friends or complain about on social media. They're tangible, often shared experiences that we can point to and say, "That! That's what's stressing me out!"

Internal Stressors

Now, internal stressors are the stressors that come from within ourselves—our thoughts, feelings, and behaviors.

Common internal stressors include:

- Negative self-talk and self-criticism
- Perfectionism and setting unrealistic expectations for yourself
- Pessimistic thinking patterns
- Fear of failure or fear of success
- Guilt or shame about past events
- Insecurity and low self-esteem
- Uncertainty about the future or major life decisions
- Feeling a lack of control over your life
- Unresolved emotional issues or trauma

- Difficulty with time management or procrastination

Internal stressors can be trickier to identify and address because they're often deeply ingrained in our thought patterns and beliefs. They're the stressors that keep us up at night, replaying conversations in our heads or worrying about things that might never happen. Understanding both types of stressors helps us recognize what's triggering our stress response. Once we can identify our stressors, we're better equipped to develop strategies to manage them—whether that's through changing our circumstances, adjusting our thought patterns, or using techniques like somatic exercises to release the tension these stressors create in our bodies.

Techniques for Identifying Your Personal Stressors

There are various techniques that you can use to piece together clues, notice patterns, and sometimes catch yourself in the act of getting stressed. They require some work and for you to be deliberate in your practice, but they certainly work:

The Body Scan Method

Your body often knows you're stressed before your mind does. Try this:

- Set aside a few minutes each day to mentally scan your body from head to toe.
- Notice any areas of tension, discomfort, or unusual sensations.
- Ask yourself: What was happening when I started feeling this tension? What was I thinking about?

This technique can help you connect physical stress symptoms to their triggers.

The Stress Journal

Keeping a stress journal can reveal patterns you might not otherwise notice. Here's how:

- Each day, jot down stressful incidents and your reactions to them.
- Note the time, place, people involved, and how you felt both emotionally and physically.
- After a week or two, review your entries. Look for common themes or recurring situations.

You might be surprised to find that certain people, places, or types of events consistently trigger your stress response.

The "What If" Game

Sometimes, our stress comes from worries about the future. Try this exercise:

- When you notice yourself feeling anxious, ask "What am I afraid might happen?"
- Follow each answer with another "What if that happened?" until you get to the root of fear.

This can help you identify whether you're stressing about realistic possibilities or unlikely scenarios.

The Energy Audit

Pay attention to what drains your energy and what replenishes it:

- Throughout your day, notice activities or interactions that leave you feeling tired or tense.
- Also, note what makes you feel energized or relaxed.
- At the end of the day, review your observations. The energy-drainers are likely your stressors.

The Mindful Pause

This technique helps you catch stress in the moment:

- Several times a day, especially when transitioning between activities, take a deliberate pause.
- During this pause, notice your thoughts, emotions, and physical sensations.
- If you're feeling stressed, ask yourself: What's contributing to this feeling right now?

The Trusted Friend Perspective

Sometimes, we're too close to our own situation to see it clearly. Try this:

- Describe your typical day or week to a trusted friend.
- Ask them if they notice any patterns or situations that seem to stress you out.
- Their outside perspective might highlight stressors you've been overlooking.

The Values Checklist

Stress often arises when our actions don't align with our values:

- Make a list of your core values (e.g., family, career growth, creativity, health).

- Review your daily activities and see how they align with these values.
- Notice if there are areas where you feel a mismatch. These misalignments can be significant sources of stress.

Somatic Exercises for Relaxation

Our emotional states are reflected in the body's physical patterns, and by altering these patterns through mindful movement, we influence our mental and emotional well-being. Somatic exercises for relaxation are designed to release tension, improve body awareness, and promote a state of calm and balance.

The following exercises are designed to release tension, improve body awareness, and promote a state of calm and balance. They introduce a series of somatic movements specifically tailored for relaxation, they are gentle, accessible, and suitable for varying physical abilities.

Standing Wall Roll Down

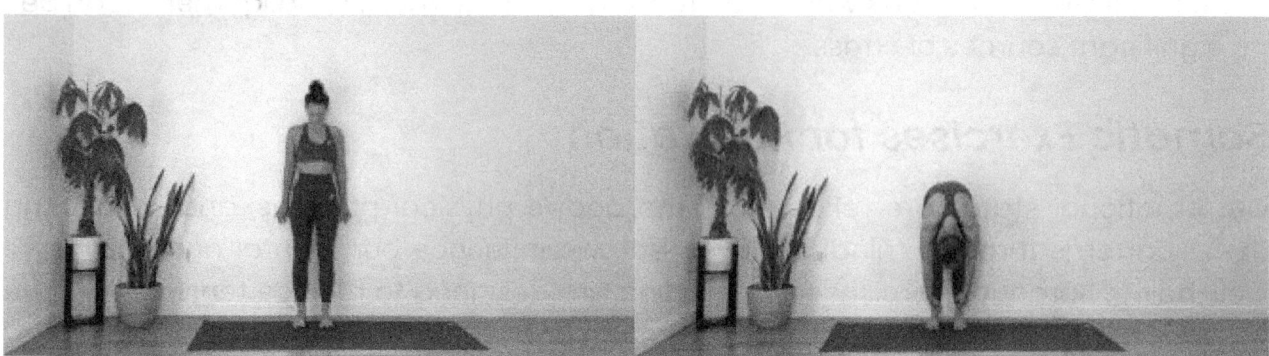

This exercise promotes spinal flexibility, releases tension in the back muscles, and encourages a connection between breath and movement. It enhances body awareness and can help improve posture.

1. Stand with your back against a wall, feet hip-width apart and about 6 inches away from the wall.

2. Begin with your entire back, shoulders, and head touching the wall.

3. Take a deep breath in. As you exhale, slowly tuck your chin to your chest and begin to peel your spine away from the wall, vertebra by vertebra.

4. Continue rolling down until your upper body is hanging towards the floor, or as far as is comfortable for you.

5. Pause for a moment, allowing your spine and back muscles to relax.

6. Inhale and begin to slowly roll back up, stacking each vertebra against the wall until you're fully upright.

7. Once upright, take a deep breath and feel the length in your spine.

8. Repeat this movement 5-10 times, moving slowly and mindfully with your breath

Supine Arm Circles

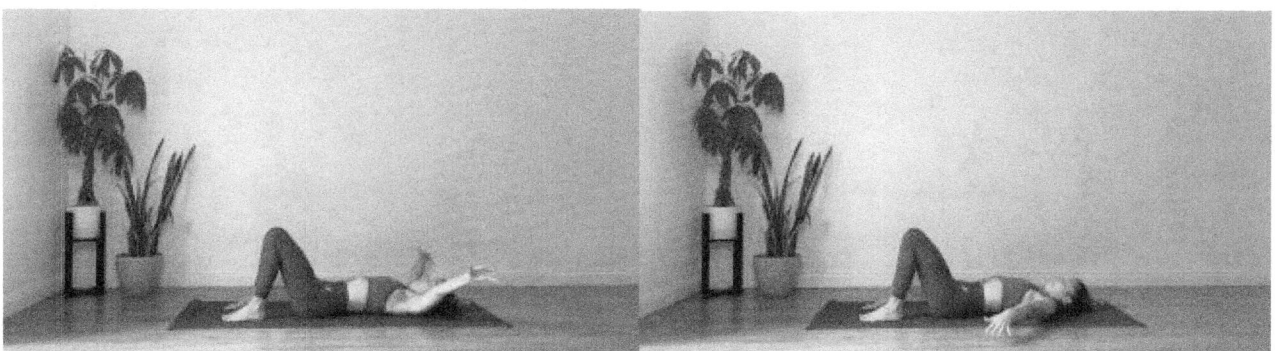

(this, but lying down)

These help release tension in the shoulders and upper back while promoting relaxation through gentle, rhythmic movement. This exercise encourages improved circulation and increased range of motion in the shoulder joints.

1. Lie on your back with your knees bent and feet flat on the floor.

2. Extend your arms out to the sides, forming a T-shape with your body.

3. Make small circular motions with your arms, keeping them in contact with the floor.

4. Gradually increase the size of the circles, but only to a comfortable range.

5. After 5-10 circles in one direction, reverse the direction.

6. Focus on your breath, inhaling as your arms move up, exhaling as they move down.

7. Continue for 1-2 minutes or for as long as comfortable.

Somatic Sunbird Pose

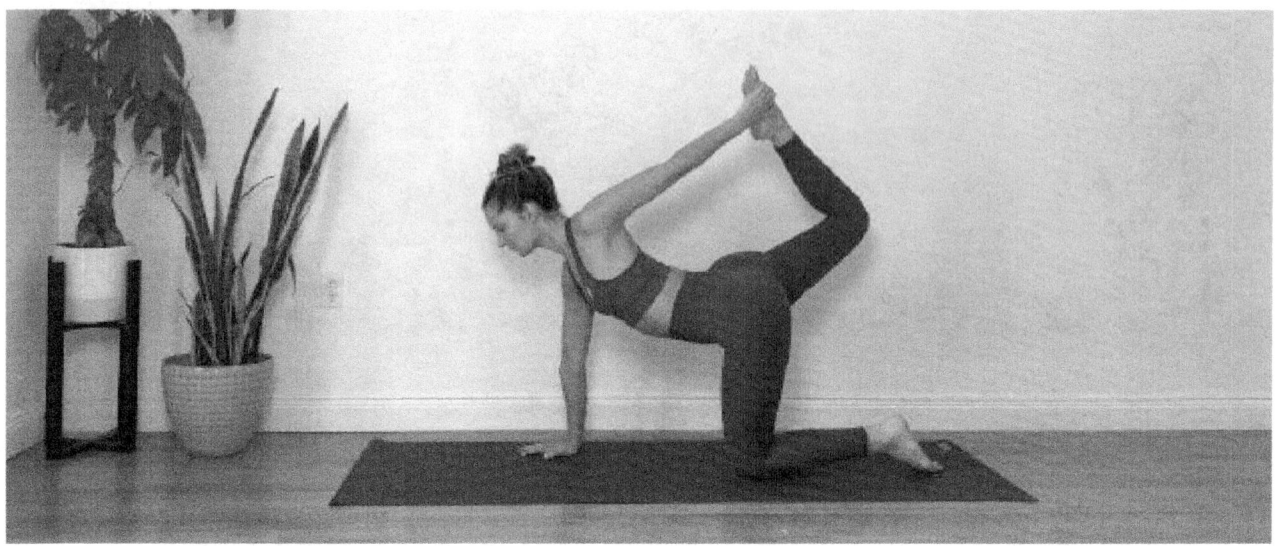

The Somatic Sunbird Pose is a progression of Bird Dog. It improves balance, strengthens the core, and enhances body awareness. This exercise promotes coordination between the upper and lower body while encouraging a focus on stability and controlled movement.

1. Start on your hands and knees in the tabletop position, with wrists under shoulders and knees under hips.

2. Slowly extend your right arm forward while simultaneously extending your left leg backward.

3. Focus on maintaining balance and keeping your spine neutral. Avoid arching your back or rotating your hips.

4. Hold this position for 3-5 breaths, focusing on stability and the sensation in your extended limbs.

5. Slowly return to the starting position.

6. Repeat on the other side, extending your left arm and right leg.

7. Alternate sides for 5-10 repetitions on each side.

Somatic Hip Rolls

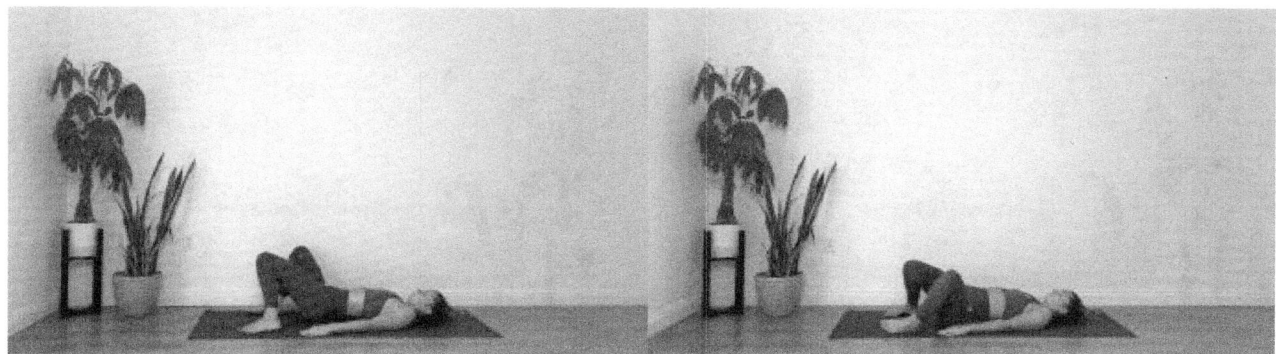

These help release tension in the lower back and hips while promoting increased awareness of the pelvic area. This gentle exercise can improve spinal mobility and encourage relaxation in the lower body.

1. Lie on your back with your knees bent and feet flat on the floor, hip-width apart.

2. Place your arms slightly out to the sides, palms down for stability.

3. Engage your core slightly to press your lower back into the floor.

4. Slowly and gently begin to roll your hips to the right, allowing your knees to lower towards the floor. Only go as far as is comfortable.

5. Pause briefly, then slowly roll your hips back to center.

6. Repeat the movement to the left side.

7. Continue alternating sides for 5-10 repetitions in each direction.

8. Focus on the sensation of your hips and lower back as you move, noticing any areas of tension or release.

Lying Hip Release

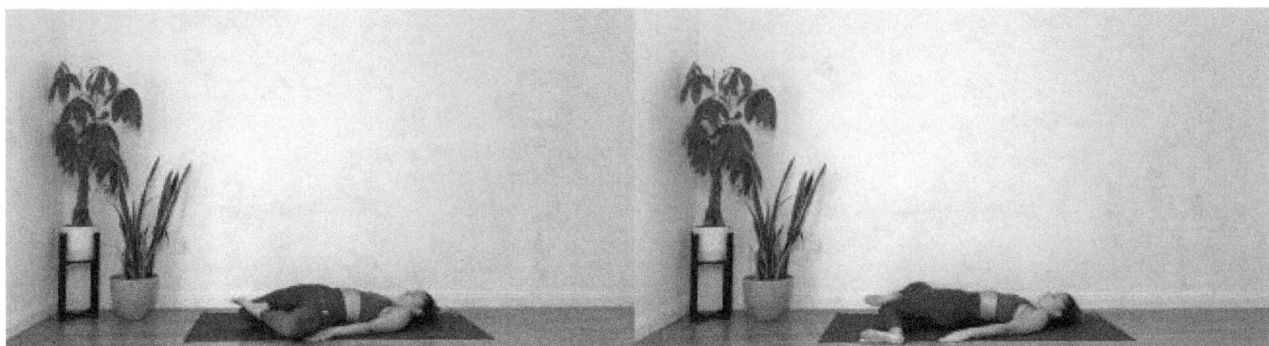

This exercise gently releases tension in the hips and lower back, promoting relaxation and increased awareness of the pelvic area.

1. Lie on your back with your knees bent and feet flat on the floor, hip-width apart.

2. Place your arms at your sides, palms down.

3. Gently allow your knees to fall to one side, keeping your feet on the floor.

4. Hold for 5-10 breaths, focusing on the stretch in your hip and lower back.

5. Slowly return to the center and repeat on the other side.

6. Continue alternating sides for 3-5 repetitions on each side.

Somatic Wave

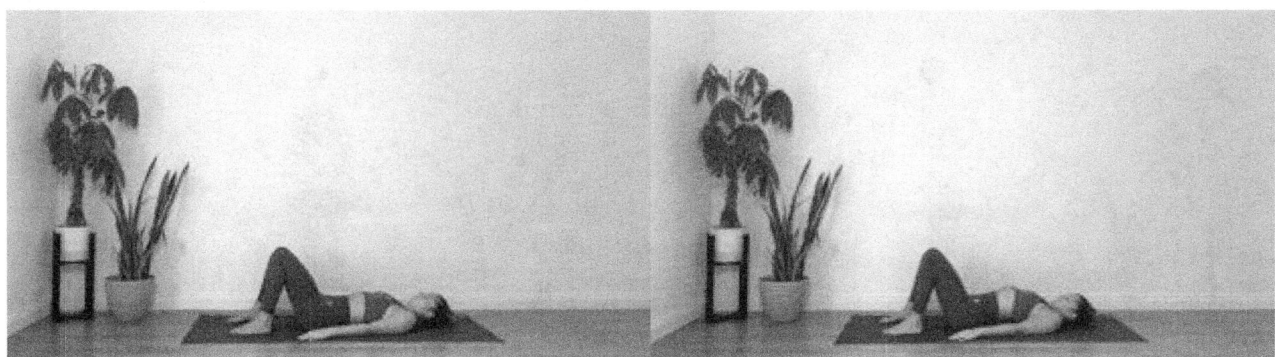

The somatic wave promotes spinal flexibility and core awareness, encouraging a fluid, wave-like movement through the spine.

1. Lie on your back with your knees bent and feet flat on the floor.

2. Begin by tucking your tailbone and rolling your spine up off the floor, vertebra by vertebra.

3. Continue rolling up until you reach your shoulder blades.

4. Pause briefly at the top, then slowly roll back down, again moving vertebrae by vertebra.

5. Focus on the sensation of each part of your spine making contact with the floor.

6. Repeat this wave-like motion 5-10 times, moving slowly and mindfully.

Standing Pelvic Tilts

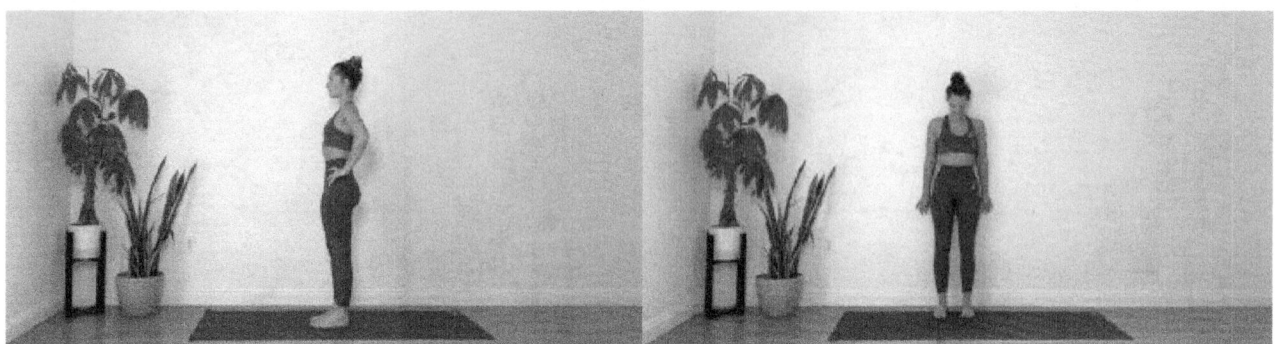

This exercise increases awareness of the pelvic position and helps release tension in the lower back.

1. Stand with your feet hip-width apart, knees slightly bent.

2. Place your hands on your hips to feel the movement.

3. Slowly tilt your pelvis forward, arching your lower back slightly.

4. Then tilt your pelvis backward, flattening your lower back.

5. Continue this gentle rocking motion, focusing on the movement of your pelvis.

6. Repeat for 10-15 cycles, coordinating the movement with your breath.

Dynamic Warrior I

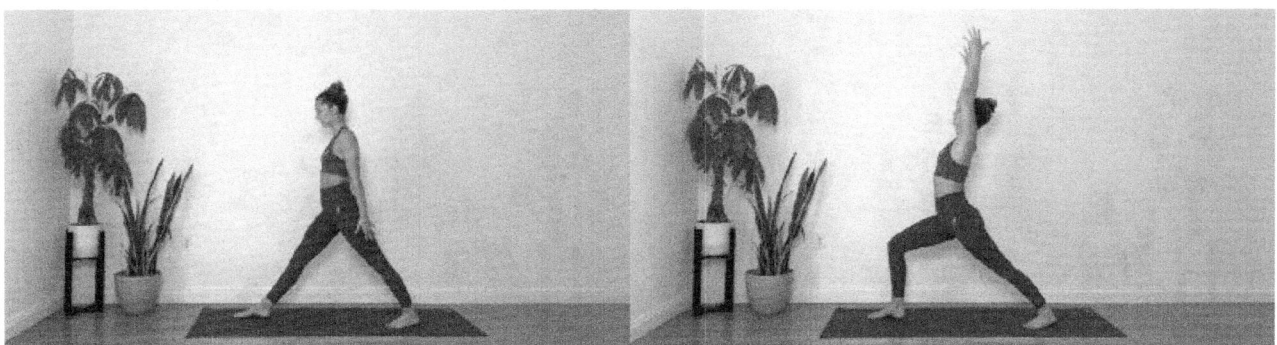

This dynamic version of the Warrior I pose promotes flexibility, balance, and body awareness.

1. Start in a standing position.

2. Step your left foot back about 3-4 feet, keeping it at a 45-degree angle.

3. Bend your right knee, aligning it over your right ankle.

4. As you inhale, raise your arms overhead, arching your back slightly.

5. As you exhale, lower your arms and straighten your front leg.

6. Continue this flowing movement, coordinating with your breath.

7. Repeat for 5-10 cycles, then switch sides.

Somatic Warrior II

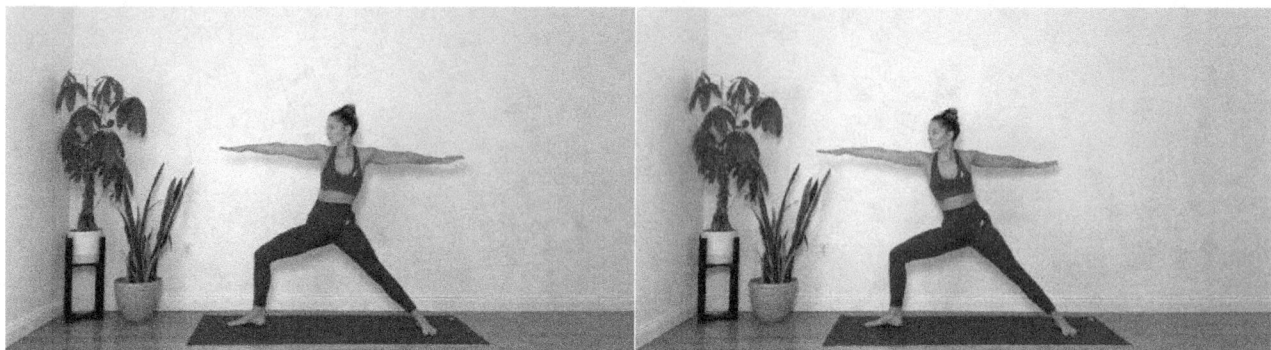

This gentle variation of Warrior II focuses on subtle movements to increase body awareness and release tension.

1. Step your feet wide apart, turning your right foot out 90 degrees and your left foot in slightly.

2. Bend your right knee, keeping it aligned over your ankle.

3. Extend your arms out to the sides at shoulder height.

4. Gently sway your upper body from side to side, feeling the weight shift in your legs.

5. Focus on the sensations in your legs, hips, and shoulders as you move.

6. Continue for 30-60 seconds, then switch sides.

Gentle Standing Twists

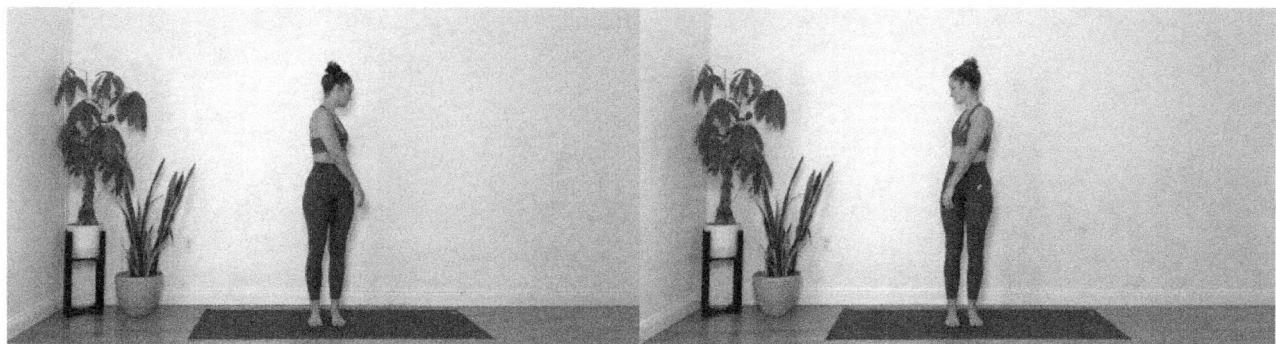

Standing twists promote spinal mobility and help release tension in the back and abdomen.

1. Stand with your feet hip-width apart, knees slightly bent.

2. Let your arms hang loosely at your sides.

3. Gently twist your upper body to the right, allowing your arms to swing naturally.

4. Then twist to the left, again letting your arms follow the movement.

5. Keep the movement slow and gentle, focusing on the sensation of the twist through your spine.

6. Repeat for 10-15 cycles, coordinating the movement with your breath.

Dynamic Tree Pose

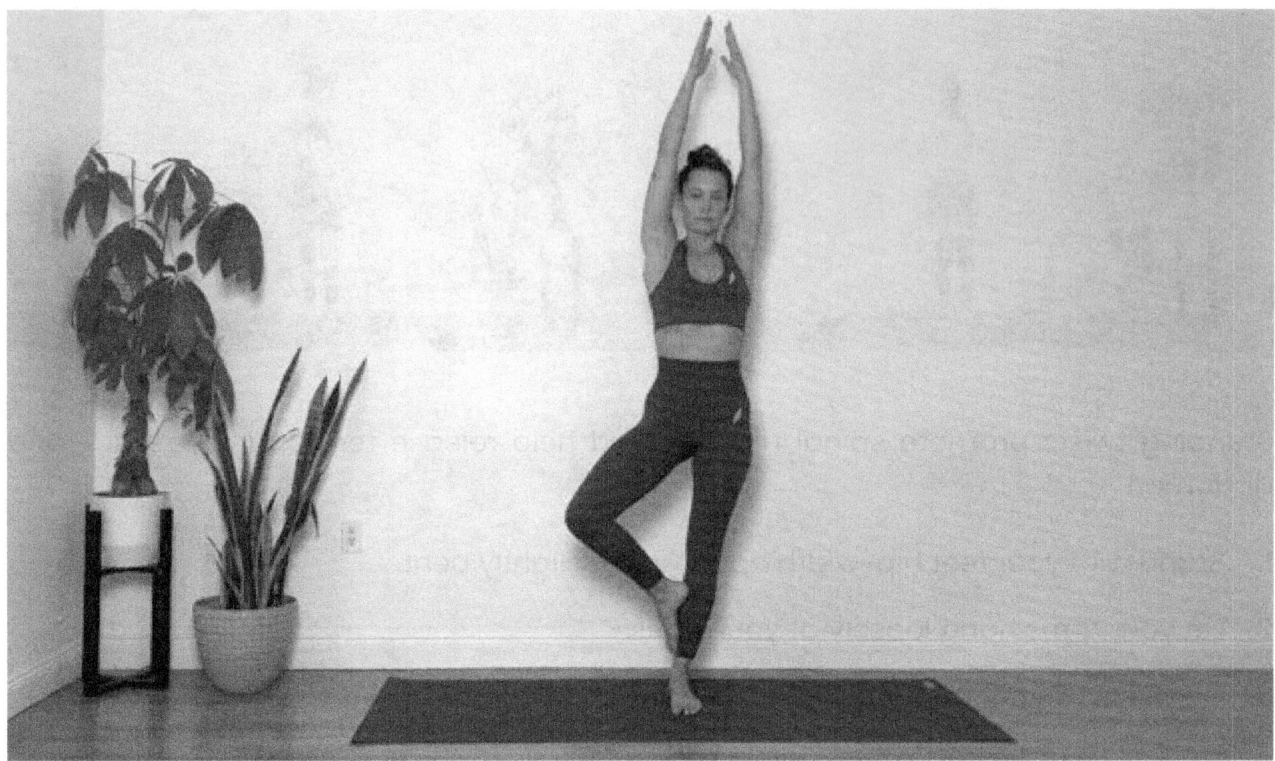

This dynamic version of Tree Pose improves balance, focus, and body awareness.

1. Stand on your left leg, bringing your right foot to rest on your left inner thigh or calf (avoid the knee).

2. As you inhale, raise your arms overhead, growing tall like a tree.

3. As you exhale, lower your arms and your right foot, returning to standing.

4. Repeat this flowing movement 5-10 times on each side.

5. Focus on maintaining balance and the sensation of grounding through your standing leg.

Somatic Forward Fold

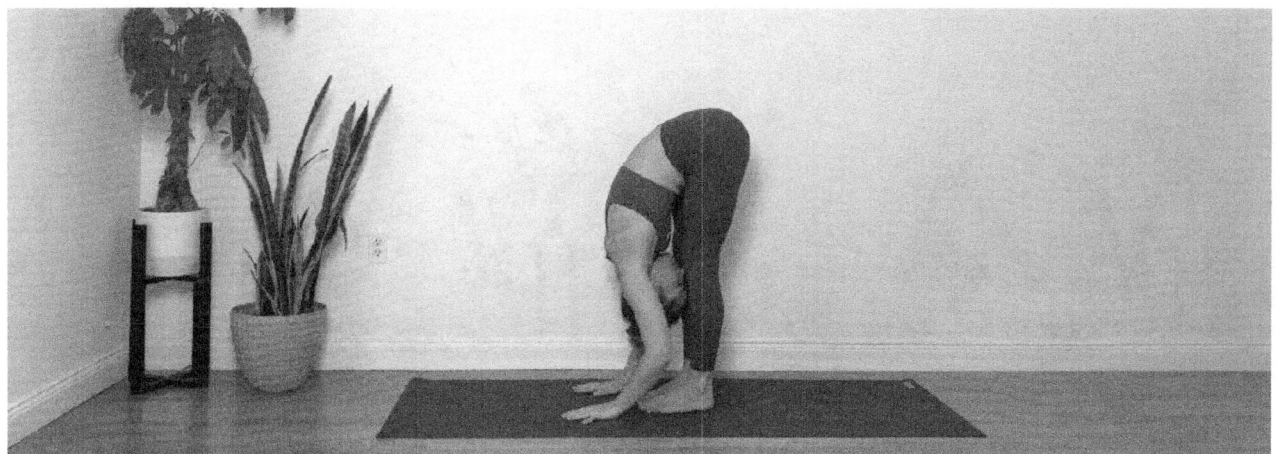

This exercise promotes flexibility in the spine and hamstrings while encouraging a sense of release and letting go.

1. Stand with your feet hip-width apart, knees slightly bent.

2. Inhale deeply, lifting your arms overhead.

3. As you exhale, slowly fold forward from your hips, allowing your arms and head to hang heavy.

4. Let your upper body relax, feeling the stretch in your back and legs.

5. Inhale and slowly roll up, stacking one vertebra at a time, until you're standing upright.

6. Repeat this flowing movement 5-7 times, moving slowly and mindfully.

Chair Pose with Arm Waves

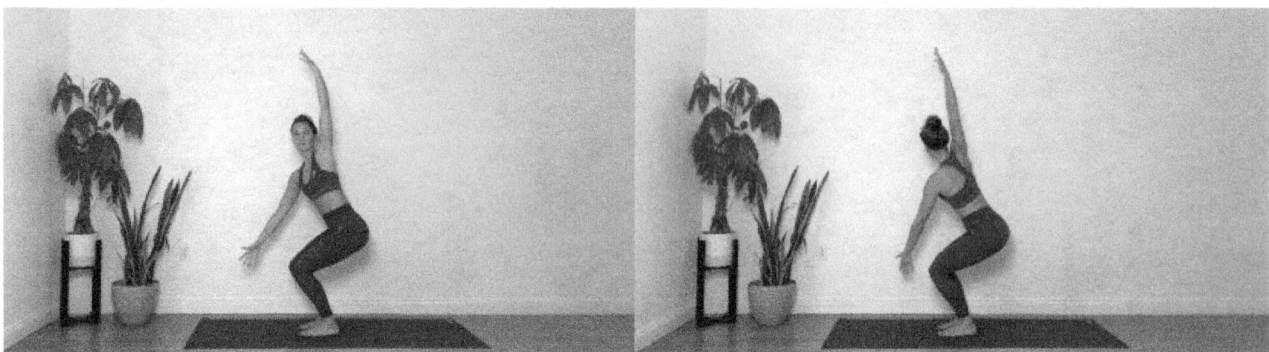

This exercise combines the grounding effect of Chair Pose with flowing arm movements to promote balance and release upper body tension.

1. Stand with your feet hip-width apart.

2. Bend your knees and lower your hips as if sitting back in a chair.

3. Raise your arms overhead.

4. While holding the chair position, begin to move your arms in a wavelike motion.

5. Allow one arm to lower as the other rises, creating a continuous, flowing movement.

6. Continue for 30-60 seconds, focusing on your breath and the sensation in your arms and legs.

Somatic Side Stretch

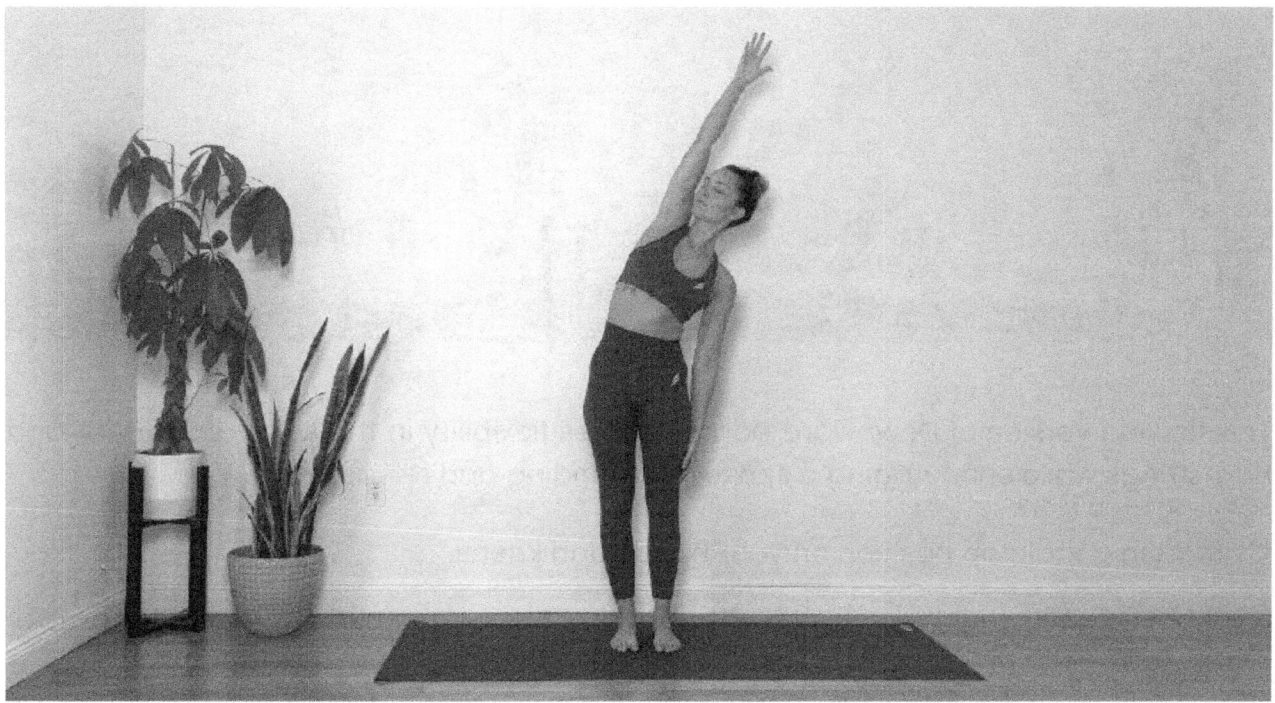

This exercise promotes lateral flexibility in the spine and ribcage, encouraging deep breathing and release of tension in the side body.

1. Stand with your feet hip-width apart.

2. Raise your right arm overhead, keeping your left arm at your side.

3. Gently lean to the left, feeling a stretch along your right side.

4. Hold for 2-3 breaths, then slowly return to center.

5. Repeat on the other side, raising your left arm and leaning to the right.

6. Continue alternating sides for 5-7 repetitions on each side.

Dynamic Downward Dog

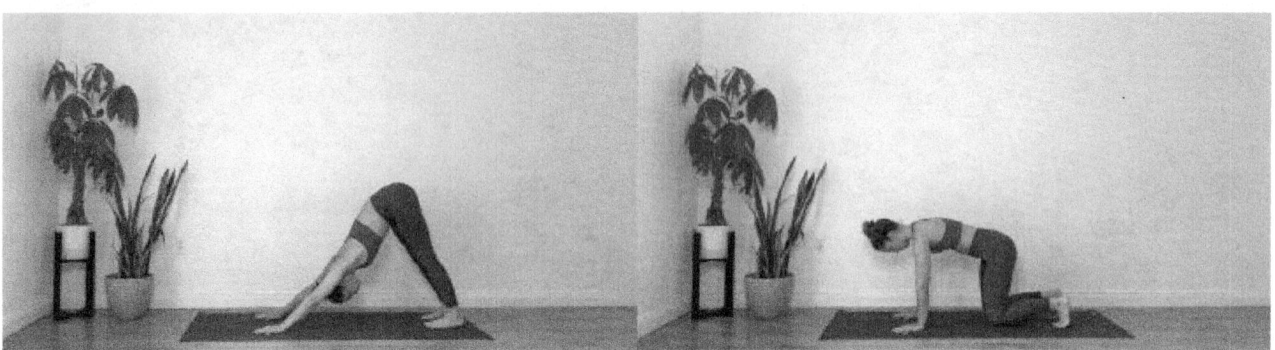

This flowing version of Downward Dog promotes flexibility in the spine, shoulders, and hamstrings while encouraging a sense of grounding and release.

1. Start in a tabletop position on your hands and knees.

2. Exhale and lift your hips, straightening your arms and legs to come into Downward Dog.

3. Hold for one breath, feeling the stretch in your back and legs.

4. Inhale and lower your hips back to the tabletop position.

5. Continue this flowing movement between tabletop and Downward Dog for 5-7 cycles.

6. Focus on the sensation of lengthening and releasing with each movement.

Somatic Crescent Lunge

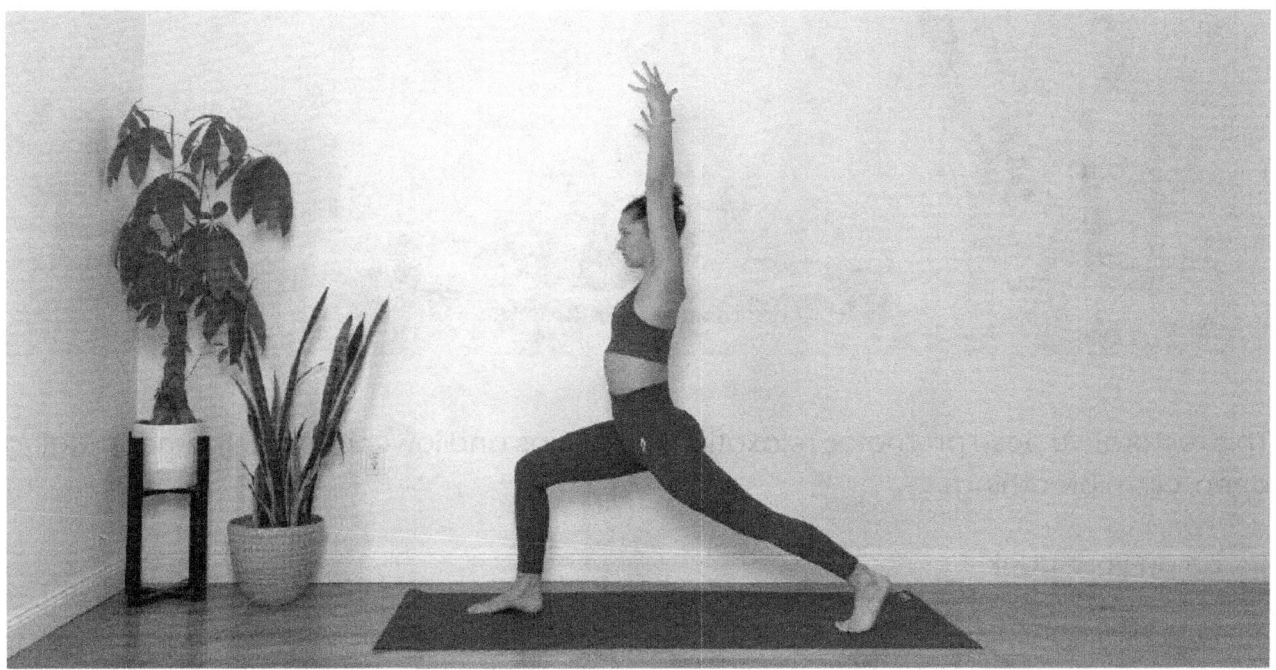

This gentle variation of Crescent Lunge promotes hip flexibility and balance while encouraging mindful movement.

1. Start in a standing position.

2. Step your right foot back into a lunge position, keeping your left knee over your left ankle.

3. Raise your arms overhead.

4. Gently sway your upper body from side to side, feeling the shift in your hips and legs.

5. After 5-7 sways, pulse up and down slightly in the lunge, moving just an inch or two.

6. Continue for 30-60 seconds, then switch sides.

Reclined Butterfly Pose

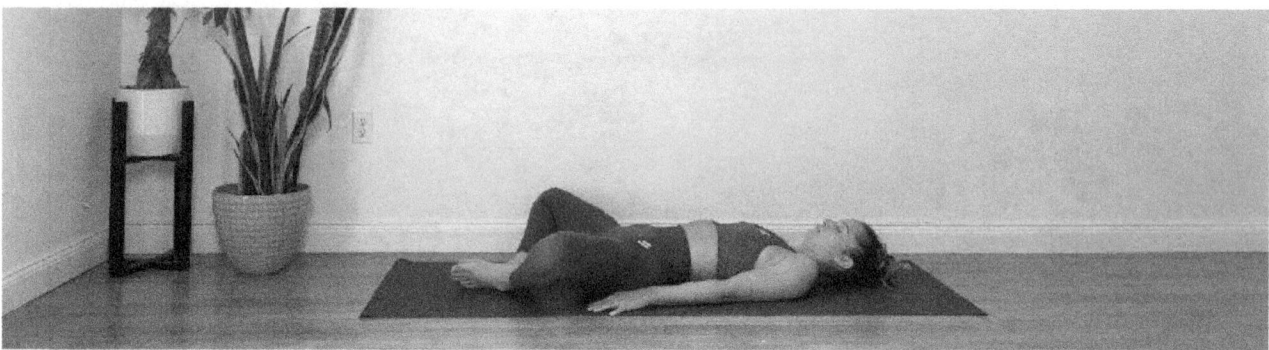

This restorative pose promotes relaxation in the hips and lower back while encouraging deep, calm breathing.

1. Lie on your back.

2. Bring the soles of your feet together, allowing your knees to fall out to the sides.

3. Place your arms at your sides, palms facing up.

4. Close your eyes and focus on your breath, feeling your belly rise and fall.

5. Gently press your lower back into the floor, then release, creating a subtle rocking motion.

6. Continue this gentle movement for 1-2 minutes, or hold the static pose for 3-5 minutes for deeper relaxation.

Meditation and Mindfulness Practices

We meditate and engage in mindfulness practices because it's how we teach our bodies to be at peace with uncertainty. These practices serve as an anchor that helps us cultivate a sense of inner calm that isn't dependent on external circumstances. They teach us to observe our thoughts and feelings without getting caught up in them, to breathe through discomfort rather than resist it, and to find moments of stillness amidst the chaos of daily life; through them, we develop a more compassionate relationship with ourselves and a more grounded approach to life's challenges.

We do get various kinds of meditation techniques, which all work a different way, these are the main ones that we usually work with for stress relief:

1. **Mindfulness Meditation:** This technique involves focusing on the present moment, typically by paying attention to your breath or bodily sensations. It's about observing your thoughts and feelings without judgment, allowing them to pass without getting caught up in them. Mindfulness meditation can help reduce stress, improve focus, and increase self-awareness.

2. **Loving-Kindness Meditation (Metta):** This practice involves cultivating feelings of love, kindness, and compassion towards yourself and others. It typically uses visualization and silent repetition of phrases. Loving-kindness meditation can help reduce negative emotions, increase positive emotions, and improve relationships.

3. **Body Scan Meditation:** This technique involves systematically focusing your attention on different parts of your body, from your toes to the top of your head. It helps increase body awareness, release physical tension, and promote relaxation. Body scan meditation can be particularly helpful for those who hold stress in their bodies or have trouble sleeping.

Mindfulness Meditation

Instructions:

1. Find a comfortable seated position. This can be on a chair or cushion, with your back straight but not rigid.

2. Close your eyes or lower your gaze.

3. Take a few deep breaths to settle into your body and the present moment.

4. Bring your attention to your breath. Notice the sensation of the breath entering and leaving your body.

5. As you breathe naturally, focus on the rise and fall of your abdomen or the feeling

of air passing through your nostrils.

6. When you notice your mind wandering (which is normal and will happen often), gently bring your attention back to your breath without judgment.

7. Continue this practice for 5-10 minutes to start, gradually increasing the duration as you become more comfortable with the technique.

8. To end the meditation, slowly bring your awareness back to your surroundings, wiggle your fingers and toes, and open your eyes.

Loving-Kindness Meditation (Metta)

Instructions:

1. Sit with your eyes closed and take a few deep breaths to center yourself.

2. Begin by focusing on your heart center, imagining a warm, glowing light in your chest.

3. Silently repeat the following phrases to yourself:

   - "May I be happy"
   - "May I be healthy"
   - "May I be safe"
   - "May I live with ease"

4. After a few minutes, bring to mind someone you care about deeply. Visualize them and repeat the same phrases, replacing "I" with "you":

   - "May you be happy"
   - "May you be healthy"
   - "May you be safe"
   - "May you live with ease"

5. Next, think of a neutral person (someone you neither like nor dislike) and repeat the phrases for them.

6. If you feel ready, bring to mind someone you have difficulty with and offer the phrases to them.

7. Finally, extend these wishes to all beings everywhere.

8. Practice for 10-15 minutes, then slowly bring your awareness back to your surroundings.

Body Scan Meditation

Instructions:

1. Lie down on your back in a comfortable position, with your arms at your sides and palms facing up.

2. Close your eyes and take a few deep breaths to relax.

3. Begin by bringing your attention to your toes. Notice any sensations present – warmth, coolness, tingling, or perhaps no sensation at all.

4. Slowly move your attention up through your body, part by part: feet, ankles, calves, knees, thighs, hips, lower back, abdomen, chest, upper back, fingers, hands, arms, shoulders, neck, and finally, your head.

5. At each part, pause for a moment to notice any sensations present. If you notice any tension, imagine breathing into that area and allowing it to soften and release.

6. If your mind wanders, gently bring your focus back to the part of the body you're currently on.

7. Once you've scanned your entire body, take a moment to notice how your body feels as a whole.

8. To end the meditation, slowly wiggle your fingers and toes, take a deep breath, and open your eyes.

9. Start with 10-15 minutes and gradually increase the duration as you become more comfortable with the practice.

Chapter 6: Tension Release and Trauma Management Exercises

Trauma is not what happens to you, it's what happens inside you as a result of what happened to you.—Gabor Maté

I was talking to a somatic therapist; we talked about a lot of things, but what stuck with me was how she articulated the idea that we can't heal in the same environments that made us "sick". Right then and there, I started to understand that "environment" isn't just about physical spaces, it also consists of the internal landscape we carry within us—our thoughts, our reactions, the tension in our muscles, the patterns of our breath. These internal environments, shaped by our experiences and especially by our traumas, can keep us locked in cycles of stress and pain long after the initial events have passed.

The answer lies in our ability to reshape our internal landscape. Through mindful movement and focused awareness that help us create new patterns of being that shift us out of traumatic holding patterns, movements that invite us into our bodies—to release, to soften, to feel safe again. Each time you practice, I want you to remember that you're laying down new neural pathways, teaching your body new ways of being. You're slowly, steadily creating an internal environment where healing isn't just possible—it's inevitable.

Why Tension Occurs

Tension is physical and emotional strain, our body's natural response to stress, perceived threats, or challenging situations. When we are stressed, our nervous system triggers a series of responses, including muscle contraction, increased heart rate, and heightened alertness. This tension serves a protective function and prepares us for action in the face of potential danger.

When we experience a traumatic event, our body's stress response is activated intensely, and if the trauma is severe or prolonged, or if we're unable to fully process the experience, this state of high alert can become chronic. The body, in an attempt to protect itself from further harm, may hold onto this tension, creating patterns of chronic muscle tightness, restricted breathing, and heightened nervous system reactivity. This physical holding becomes a way of containing the unresolved trauma, almost as if the body is trying to create a protective armor against future threats.

If this tension remains released, it can lead to a host of physical and psychological issues; chronic muscle tension can result in pain, reduced flexibility, and even structural imbalances in the body. On a psychological level, unreleased tension can contribute to anxiety, irritability, and difficulty relaxing; over time, this state of chronic tension can dysregulate the nervous system, making it harder to return to a state of calm and potentially increasing vulnerability to stress-related health problems. Our ability to fully engage in the present moment is also deeply affected because part of our energy is constantly devoted to maintaining this state of alert readiness.

Symptoms of Tension

Tension shows up differently throughout different parts of the body and mind. Here Are some of the most common symptoms that may indicate you're experiencing tension:

Physical Symptoms:

1. Muscle tightness or stiffness, especially in the neck, shoulders, and back

2. Headaches, particularly tension headaches

3. Jaw-clenching or teeth-grinding

4. Chest tightness

5. Rapid heartbeat

6. Shallow or rapid breathing

7. Digestive issues (e.g., stomachaches, nausea, constipation, or diarrhea)

8. Fatigue or low-energy

9. Insomnia or disturbed sleep

10. Sweating, especially in the palms or armpits

11. Cold hands or feet

12. Frequent urination

13. Decreased libido

Emotional Symptoms:

1. Irritability or short temper

2. Anxiety or nervousness

3. Mood swings

4. Feeling overwhelmed

5. Depression or persistent low mood

6. Emotional numbness

7. Increased emotional reactivity

8. Difficulty feeling joy or pleasure

Cognitive Symptoms:

1. Difficulty concentrating or focusing

2. Racing thoughts

3. Forgetfulness or memory problems

4. Indecisiveness

5. Constant worrying

6. Negative self-talk

7. Difficulty in problem-solving

8. Decreased creativity

Behavioral Symptoms:

1. Procrastination or avoiding responsibilities

2. Nervous habits (e.g., nail biting, hair twirling, foot tapping)

3. Changes in appetite (eating too much or too little)

4. Increased use of alcohol, cigarettes, or drugs

5. Social withdrawal

6. Relationship conflicts

7. Decreased productivity

8. Restlessness or inability to relax

It's important to note that everyone experiences tension differently, and you may not have all these symptoms. If you're experiencing several of these symptoms persistently, it may be a sign that you're dealing with significant tension. In such cases, practicing tension-release exercises, seeking support from a mental health professional, or consulting with a healthcare provider can be beneficial.

Somatic Movement for Tension Release

Seated Forward Fold with Rocking

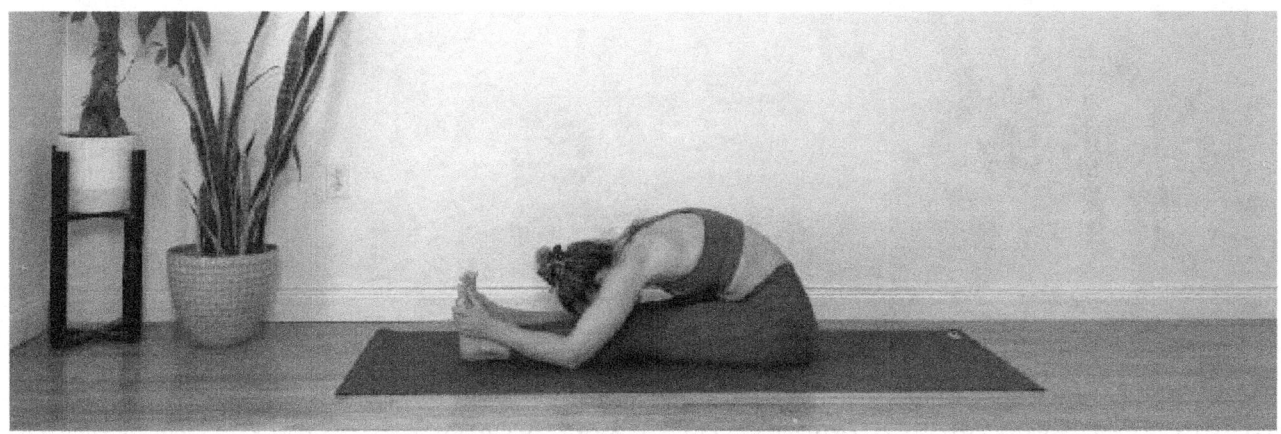

This exercise gently stretches the back muscles and promotes relaxation through a soothing rocking motion. It can help release tension in the lower back and promote a sense of grounding.

1. Sit on the floor with your legs extended in front of you.

2. Inhale deeply, lengthening your spine.

3. As you exhale, slowly fold forward from your hips, reaching towards your feet.

4. Allow your upper body to relax over your legs, letting your head hang heavy.

5. Gently rock your upper body forward and back, feeling the stretch shift in your back.

6. Continue rocking for 30-60 seconds, breathing deeply.

7. Slowly roll up to a seated position, one vertebra at a time.

Thread The Needle

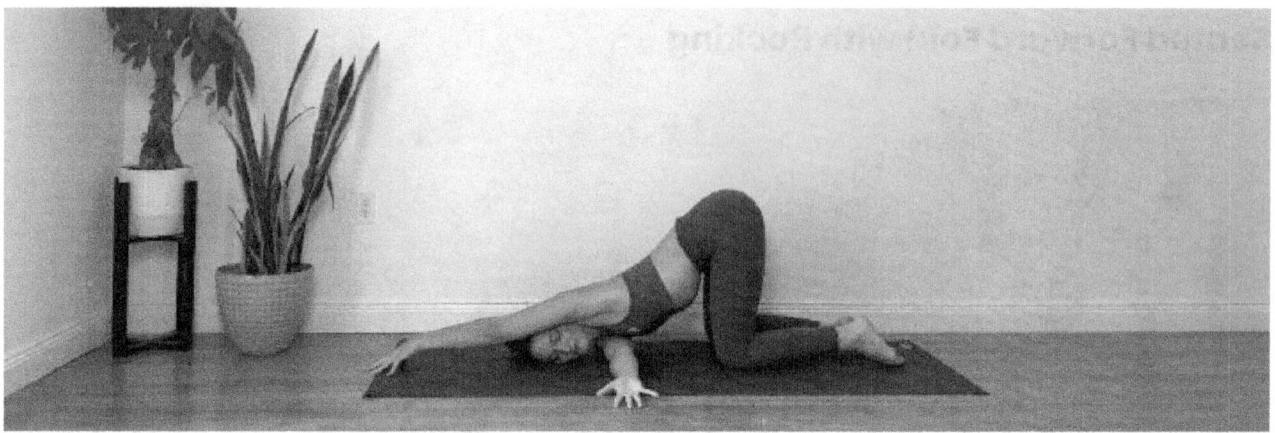

Thread the Needle offers a unique way to work on spinal mobility and upper body flexibility. It's generally accessible for most fitness levels but can be modified as needed.

1. Start on your hands and knees in a tabletop position.

2. Slide your right arm under your left arm and through the space between your left arm and left knee, as if you're threading a needle.

3. Lower your right shoulder and the right side of your head to the ground (or as close as is comfortable).

4. Keep your left hand planted on the ground for support, or for a deeper stretch, extend it forward.

5. Hold this position for 30 seconds to 1 minute, breathing deeply.

6. Slowly unwind and return to the starting position.

7. Repeat on the other side, threading your left arm under your right.

8. Do this 2-3 times on each side.

Seated Side Bend

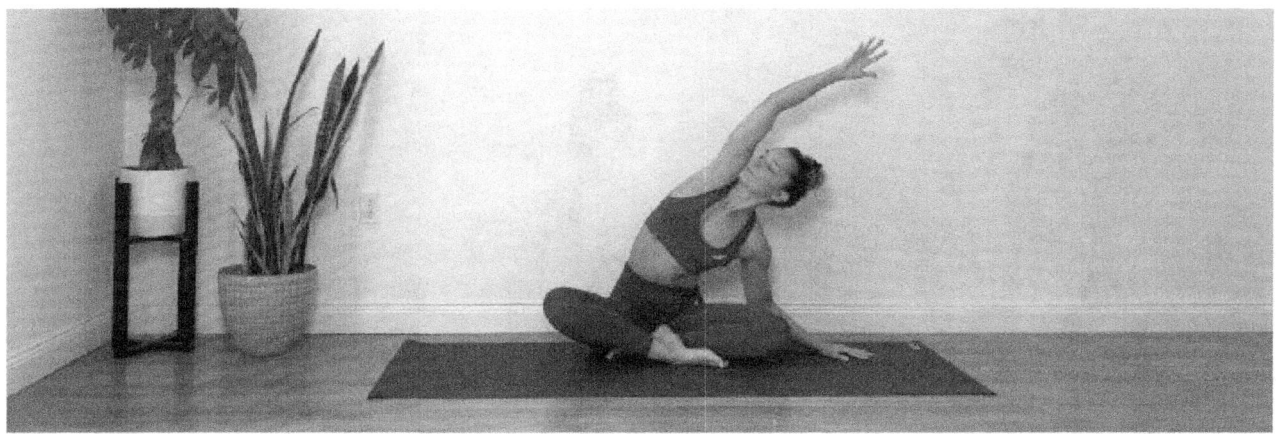

This exercise stretches the sides of the body, releasing tension in the obliques and intercostal muscles. It can help improve lateral flexibility and promote deep breathing.

1. Sit with your legs crossed or extended.

2. Extend your right arm overhead, keeping your left hand on the floor for support.

3. Inhale deeply, feeling your right side lengthen.

4. As you exhale, gently bend to the left, feeling a stretch along your right side.

5. Hold for 3-5 breaths, focusing on the sensation of lengthening.

6. Slowly return to the center and repeat on the other side.

7. Perform 3-5 side bends on each side, moving mindfully.

Seated Figure Four Stretch

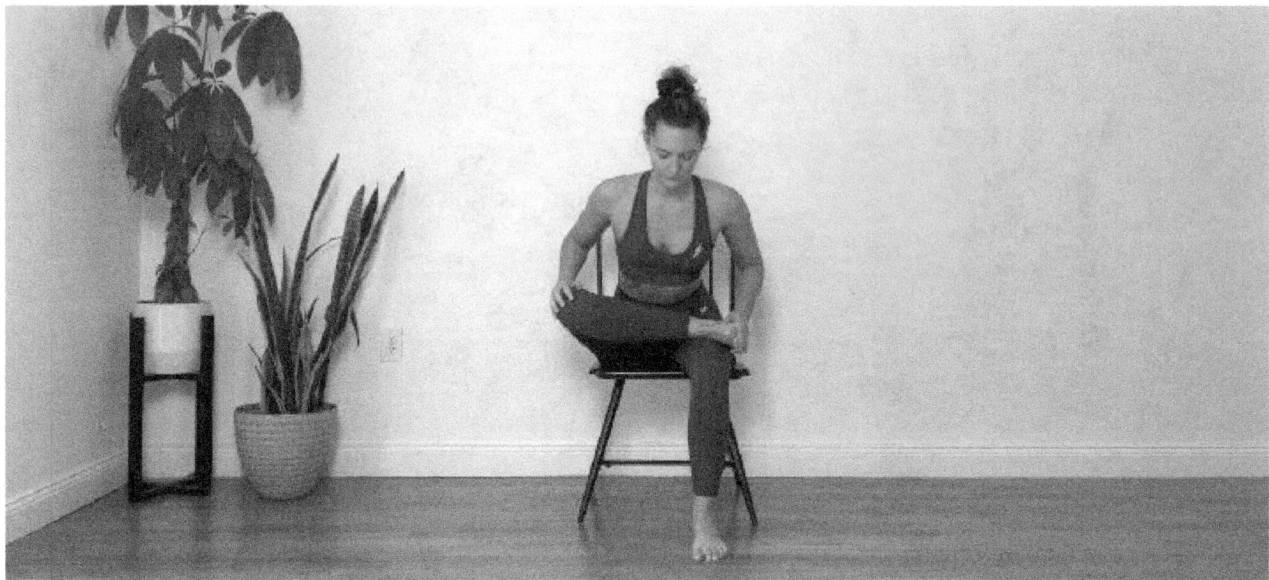

This stretch targets the hips and lower back, areas where many people hold tension. The gentle rocking motion can help release tightness and promote relaxation in these areas.

1. Sit on the edge of a chair with your feet flat on the floor.

2. Cross your right ankle over your left knee, creating a figure-four shape.

3. Flex your right foot to protect your knee.

4. Sit tall, lengthening your spine.

5. Gently lean forward, feeling a stretch in your right hip.

6. Begin a gentle rocking motion, moving slightly forward and back.

7. Continue rocking for 30-60 seconds, breathing deeply.

8. Switch legs and repeat on the other side.

Seated Arm Circles

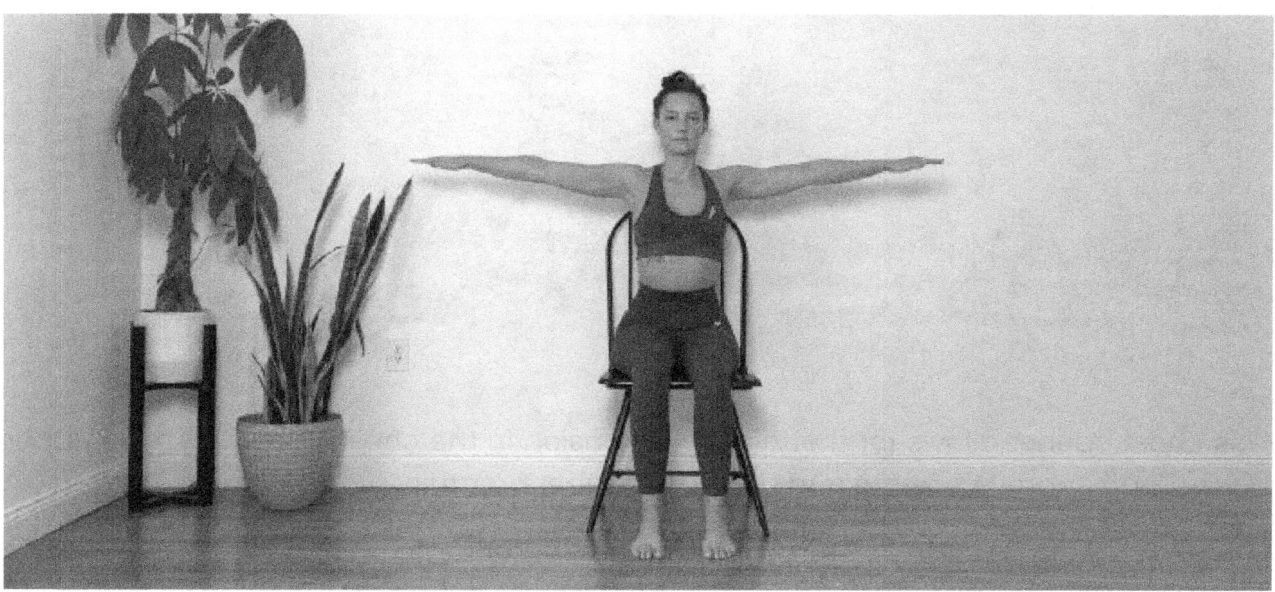

Arm circles release tension in the shoulders and upper back. The circular motion can improve shoulder mobility and promote relaxation in the upper body.

1. Sit with your spine straight and feet flat on the floor.

2. Extend your arms out to the sides at shoulder height.

3. Begin making small circular motions with your arms.

4. Gradually increase the size of the circles, but stay within a comfortable range.

5. After 30 seconds, reverse the direction of the circles.

6. Focus on your breath and the sensation in your shoulders and arms.

7. Continue for 1-2 minutes, alternating directions as desired.

Somatic Chest Opener

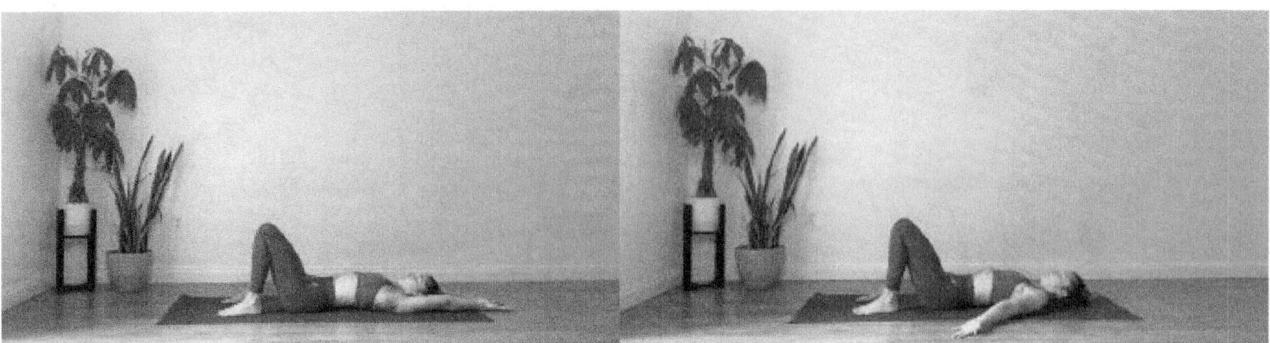

This chest opener allows for the release of tension in the chest, shoulders, and upper back. It can improve posture and promote deeper breathing.

1. Lie on your back with your knees bent and feet flat on the floor.

2. Extend your arms out to the sides, palms facing up.

3. Inhale deeply, feeling your chest expand.

4. As you exhale, gently press your arms into the floor.

5. Slowly move your arms up towards your head, then back down to your sides.

6. Focus on the stretch in your chest and the movement of your shoulder blades.

7. Repeat this movement 5-10 times, moving slowly and mindfully.

Reclined Hamstring Stretch

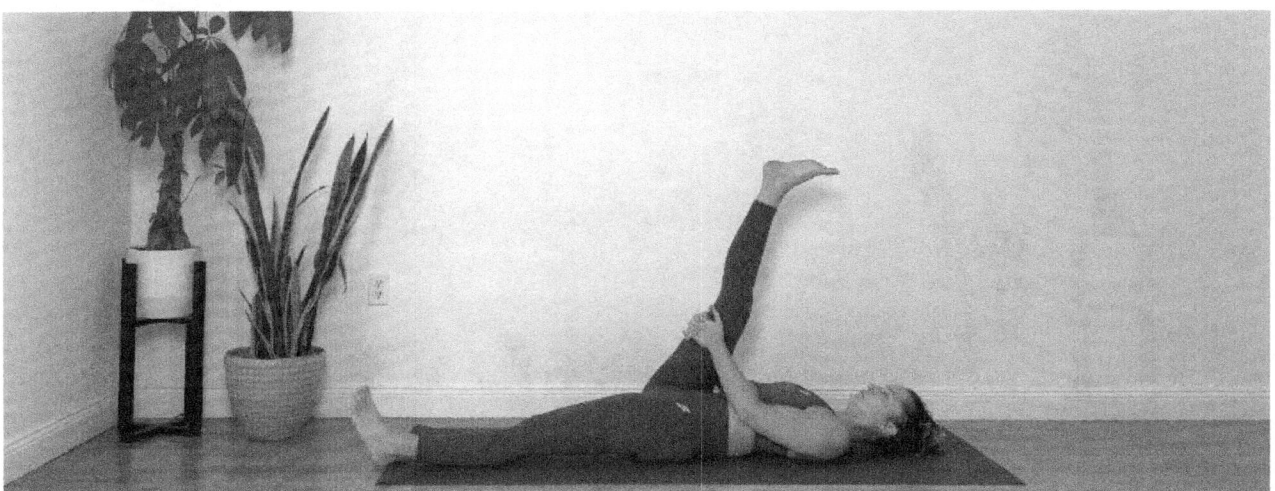

The gentle movements can improve flexibility and promote relaxation while releasing tension in the hamstrings and lower back.

1. Lie on your back with both legs extended.

2. Lift your right leg straight up towards the ceiling.

3. Place your hands behind your thigh or use a strap around your foot.

4. Gently flex and point your foot, feeling the stretch change in your hamstring.

5. Make small circles with your ankle in both directions.

6. Hold for 30-60 seconds, then slowly lower your leg.

7. Repeat with the left leg.

Somatic Frog Pose

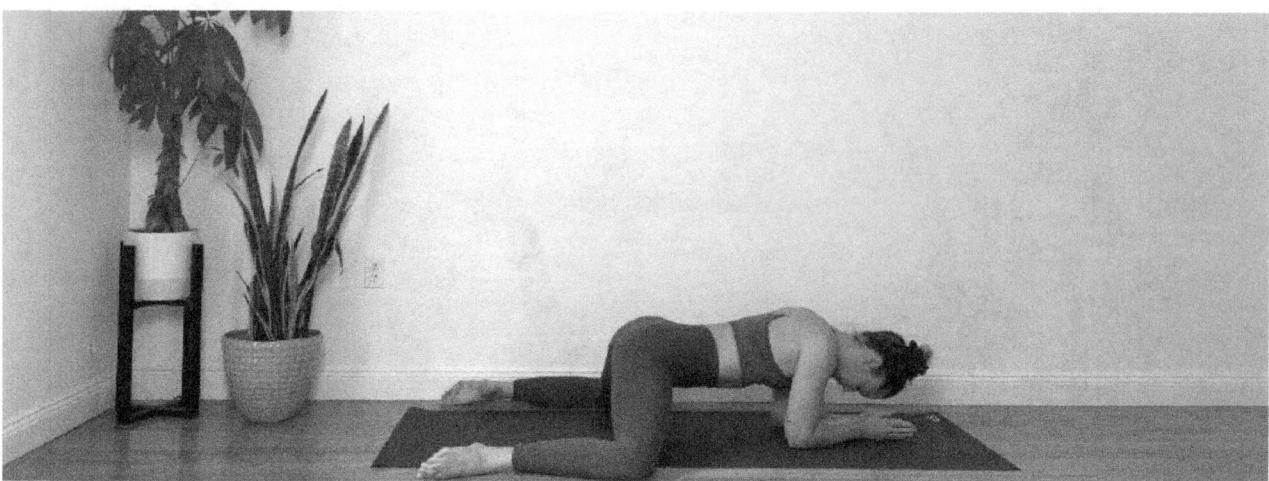

This exercise releases tension in the hips and lower back. The rocking motion can help improve hip mobility and promote relaxation.

1. Start on your hands and knees.

2. Widen your knees apart, keeping your feet together.

3. Slowly lower your upper body onto your forearms.

4. Gently rock your hips back and forth.

5. Focus on your breath and the sensation in your hips.

6. Continue rocking for 30-60 seconds.

7. Slowly return to hands and knees.

Somatic Cobra Pose

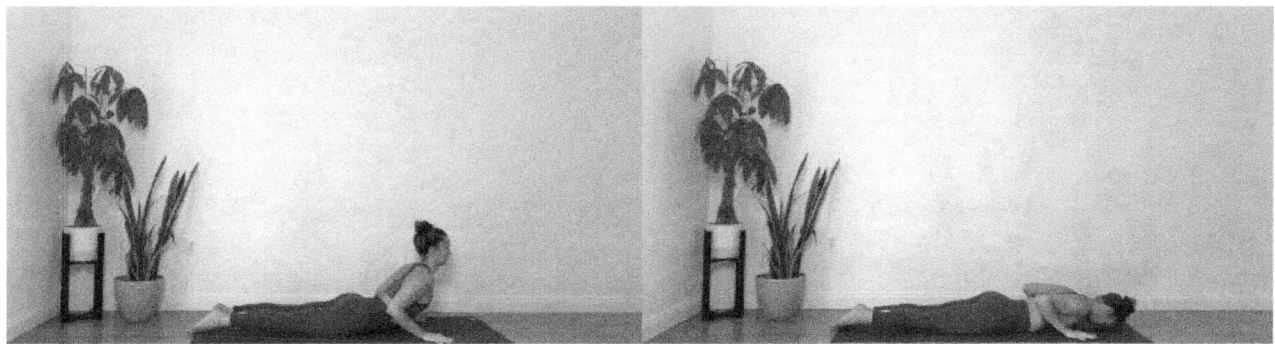

This exercise helps release tension in the spine and chest. It can improve spinal flexibility and promote better posture.

1. Lie face down with your forehead on the floor and hands by your shoulders.

2. Inhale and gently lift your chest off the floor, keeping your lower body relaxed.

3. Exhale and slowly lower back down.

4. Focus on the movement initiated from your upper back.

5. Repeat this gentle lifting and lowering 5-10 times.

6. Move slowly and mindfully, coordinating with your breath.

Somatic Half-Bow Pose

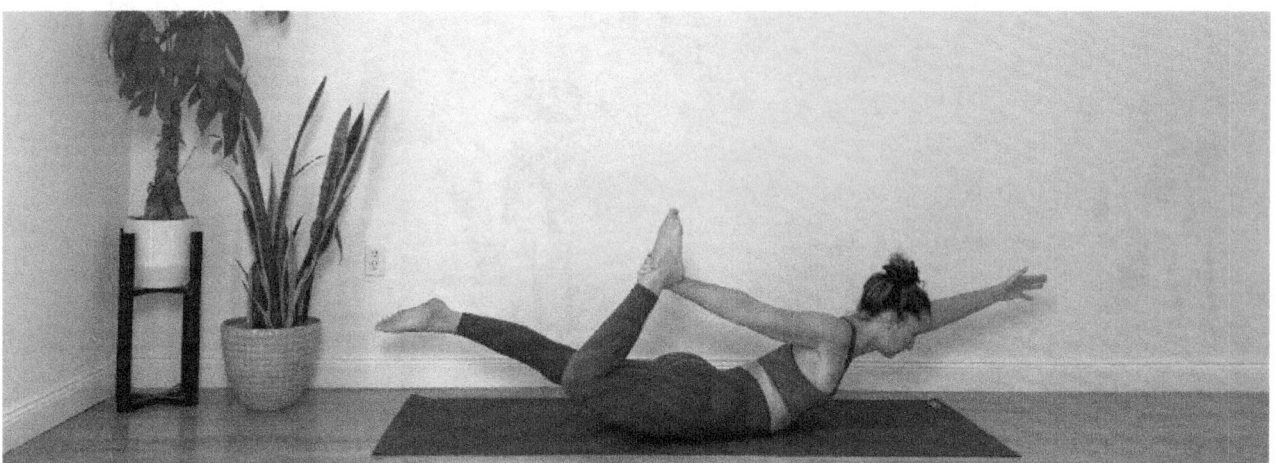

This exercise releases tension in the back, hips, and thighs. It can improve spinal mobility and hip flexibility.

1. Lie face down with your arms along your sides.

2. Bend your right knee, bringing your heel towards your buttocks.

3. Reach back with your right hand and gently grasp your right ankle.

4. Inhale and lift your right leg slightly off the floor.

5. Exhale and lower it back down.

6. Repeat this gentle lifting and lowering 5-7 times.

7. Release and switch to the left side.

Child's Pose with Arm Walks

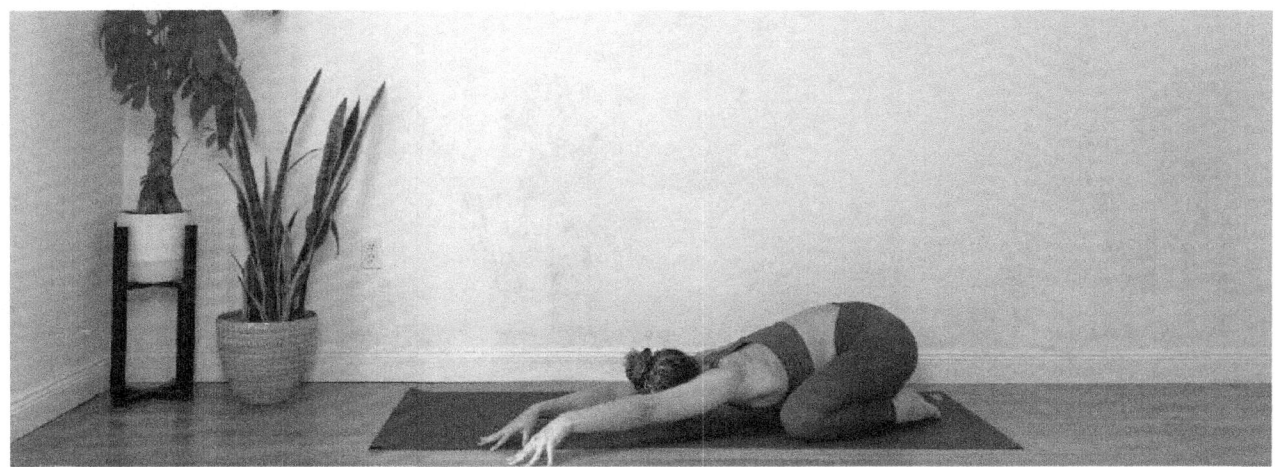

This exercise releases tension in the back, shoulders, and hips. The arm movements can provide a gentle stretch to the side body.

1. Start in Child's Pose with your knees wide and big toes touching.

2. Extend your arms out in front of you.

3. Walk your hands to the right, feeling a stretch along your left side.

4. Hold for 3-5 breaths.

5. Slowly walk your hands back to the center, then to the left side.

6. Hold for 3-5 breaths.

7. Repeat this sequence 3-5 times on each side.

Somatic Scapula Mobilization

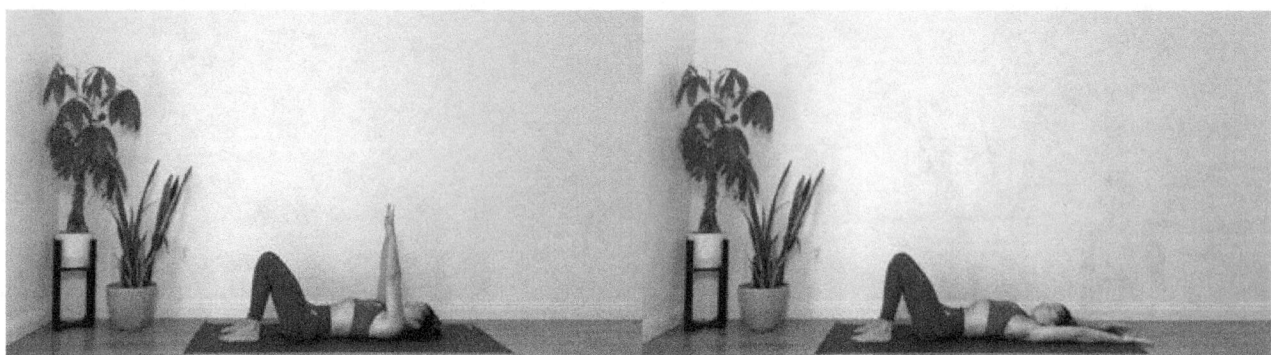

This exercise helps release tension in the shoulder blades and upper back. It can improve shoulder mobility and posture.

1. Lie on your back with your knees bent and feet flat on the floor.

2. Extend your arms towards the ceiling.

3. Slowly reach your arms up and back, as if trying to touch the floor above your head.

4. Then, bring your arms back down towards your hips.

5. Focus on the movement of your shoulder blades as you do this.

6. Repeat this movement 10-15 times, moving slowly and mindfully.

Somatic Pigeon Pose

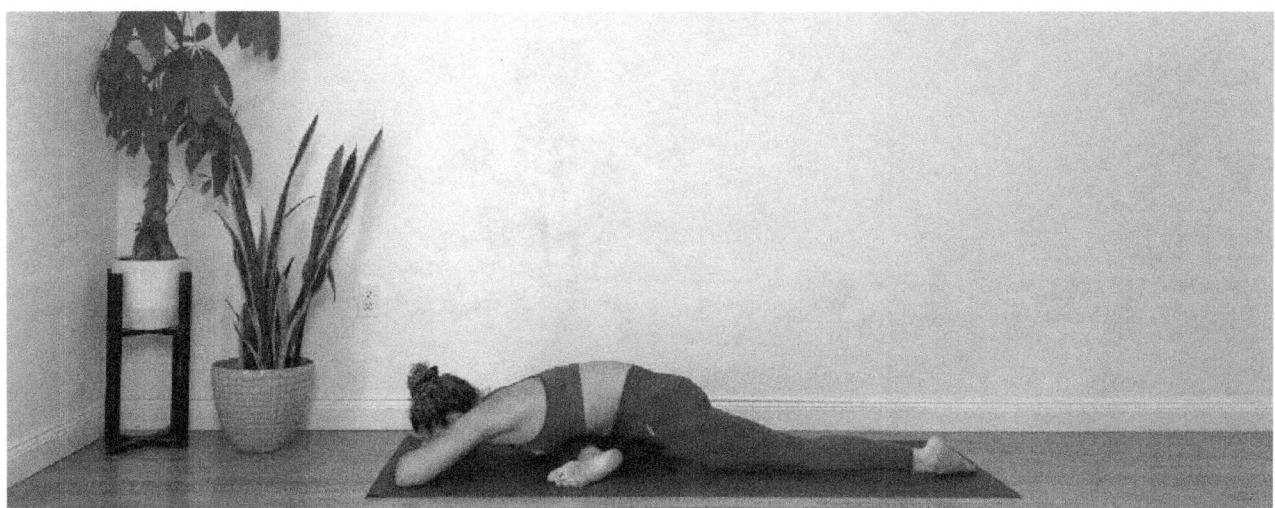

This exercise releases tension in the hips and lower back. The gentle movements can help improve hip flexibility and reduce lower back pain.

1. Start on your hands and knees.

2. Bring your right knee forward and place it behind your right wrist.

3. Extend your left leg back.

4. Lower your upper body onto your forearms or rest your forehead on the floor.

5. Gently rock your hips from side to side.

6. Focus on your breath and the sensation in your right hip.

7. Continue rocking for 30-60 seconds.

8. Slowly return to hands and knees and repeat on the other side.

Reclined Spinal Twist

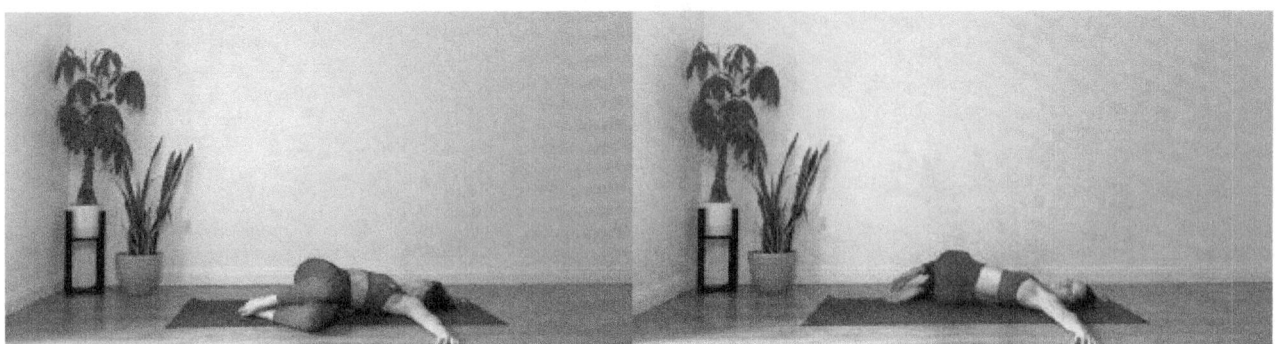

This gentle twist helps release tension in the spine, lower back, and hips. It can improve spinal mobility and promote relaxation.

Lie on your back with your knees bent and feet flat on the floor.

1. Extend your arms out to the sides in a T-shape.

2. Keeping your shoulders flat on the floor, gently lower both knees to the right side.

3. Turn your head to the left if comfortable.

4. Hold for 5-10 breaths, focusing on the sensation of lengthening through your spine.

5. Slowly bring your knees back to the center.

6. Repeat on the left side.

Dynamic Bridge Pose

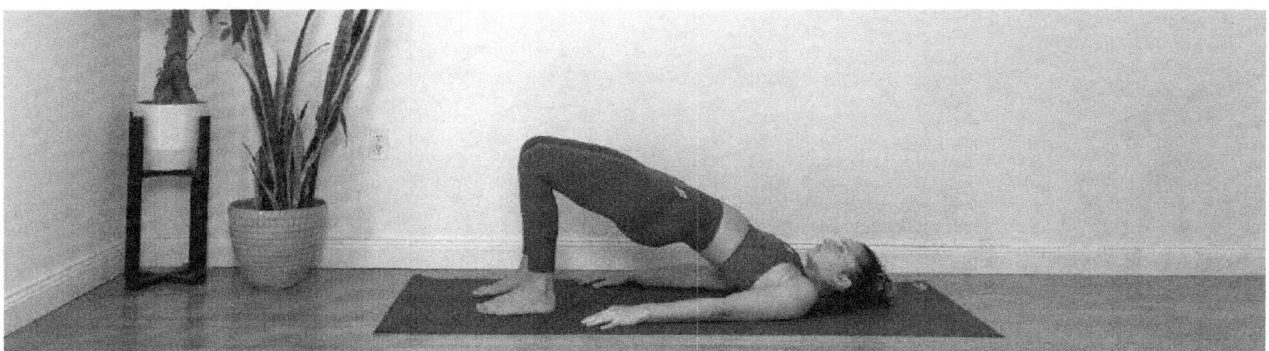

This exercise strengthens the core and lower body while releasing tension in the spine and hips. The dynamic movement can improve circulation and spinal flexibility.

1. Lie on your back with your knees bent and feet flat on the floor, hip-width apart.

2. Place your arms alongside your body, palms down.

3. Inhale and slowly lift your hips off the floor, rolling up through your spine.

4. Exhale and slowly lower back down, rolling through your spine.

5. Focus on moving one vertebra at a time, both up and down.

6. Repeat this movement 10-15 times, coordinating with your breath.

Standing Spinal Wave

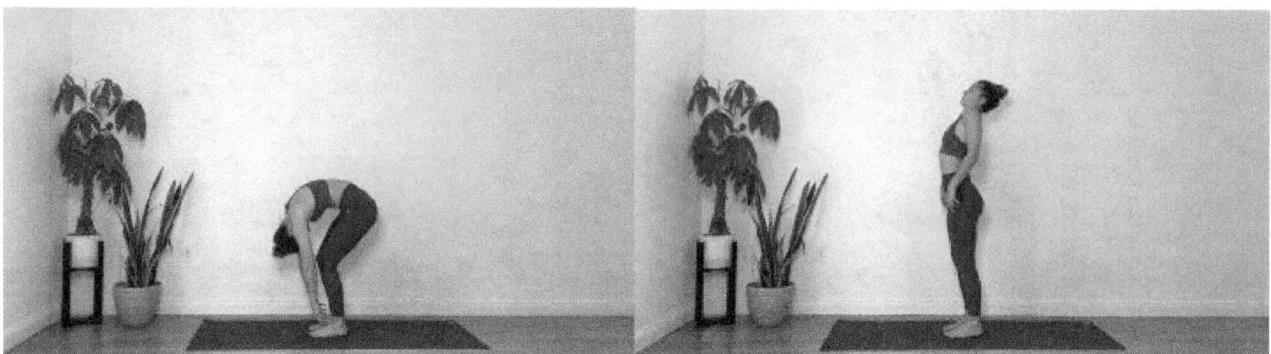

This exercise promotes flexibility in the spine, releases tension in the back and neck, and can help improve posture and body awareness.

1. Stand with your feet hip-width apart, knees slightly bent.

2. Begin by dropping your chin to your chest, then slowly roll down through your spine, vertebra by vertebra.

3. When you reach the bottom, let your upper body hang loosely for a moment.

4. Slowly begin to roll back up, starting from your tailbone and stacking each vertebra until your head is the last to come up.

5. Once upright, gently arch your back, lifting your chest and extending your spine backwards slightly.

6. From this arched position, initiate the wave again by dropping your chin to your chest.

7. Continue this fluid, wave-like motion for 1-2 minutes, focusing on moving smoothly through each part of your spine.

8. Coordinate your breath with the movement: exhale as you roll down, inhale as you roll up.

Somatic Shoulder Bridge

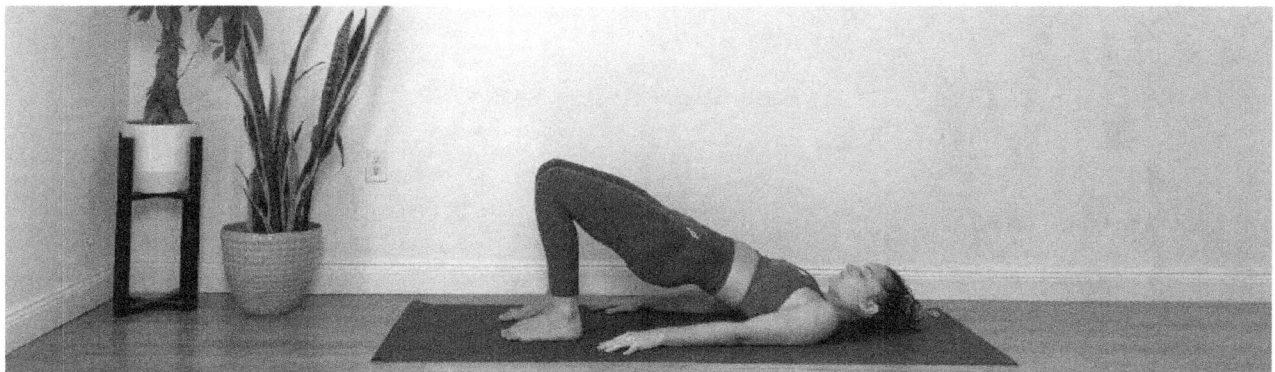

This exercise strengthens the lower body while releasing tension in the spine and hips. The dynamic movement can improve lower back flexibility and core strength.

1. Lie on your back with your knees bent and feet flat on the floor, hip-width apart.

2. Press your arms and shoulders firmly into the floor.

3. Inhale and slowly lift your hips off the floor, creating a diagonal line from knees to shoulders.

4. Exhale and slowly lower your hips back down.

5. Focus on moving one vertebra at a time, both up and down.

6. Repeat this movement 10-15 times, coordinating with your breath.

Knees to Chest Rocking

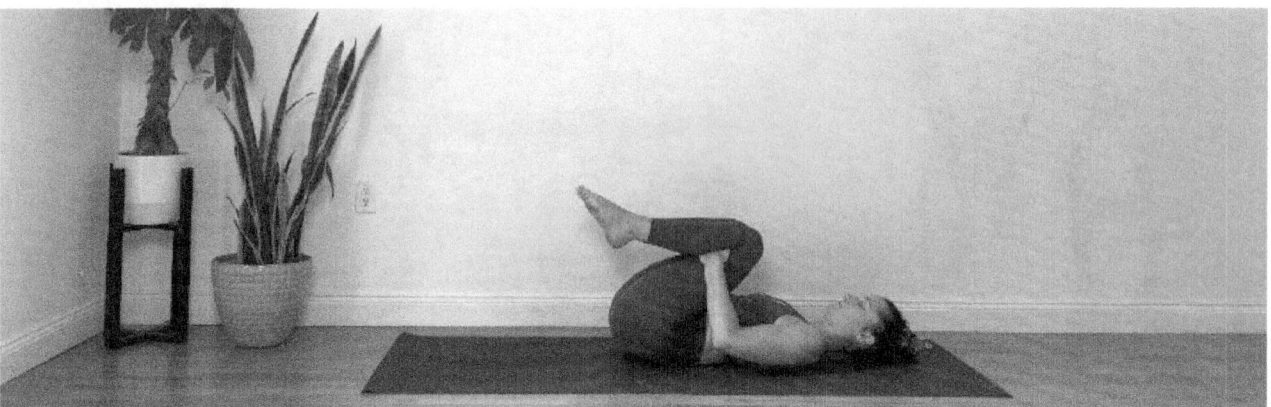

This gentle exercise releases tension in the lower back and hips. The rocking motion can promote relaxation and improve spinal mobility.

1. Lie on your back and hug your knees to your chest.

2. Wrap your arms around your shins or behind your thighs.

3. Gently rock your body from side to side.

4. Focus on the massage-like sensation on your lower back.

5. Continue rocking for 30-60 seconds, breathing deeply.

Supine Knee-to-Chest Pose (Apanasana)

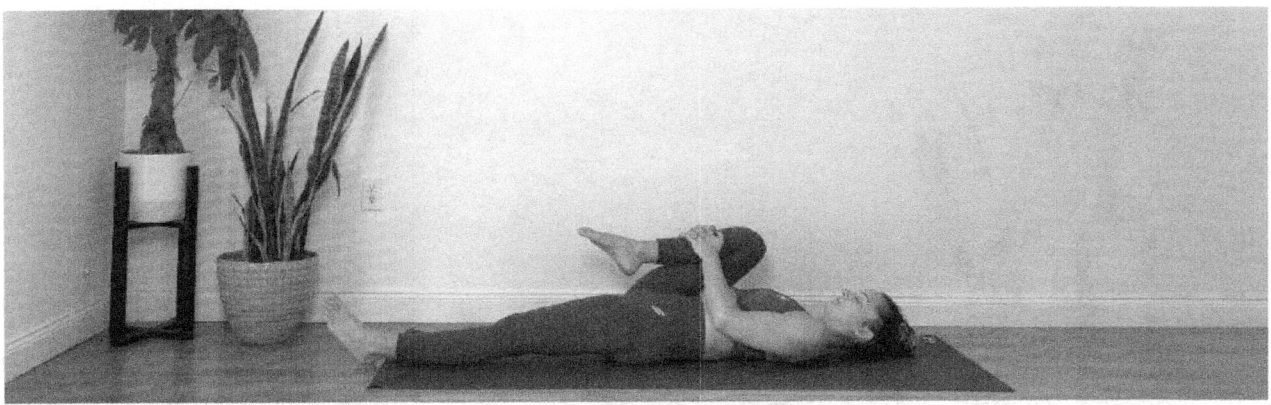

This pose helps release tension in the lower back and hips. It can aid digestion and promote overall relaxation.

1. Lie on your back with your knees bent and feet flat on the floor.

2. Bring your right knee towards your chest, holding it with both hands.

3. Keep your left foot on the floor or extend the left leg if comfortable.

4. Hold for 5-10 breaths, feeling the stretch in your lower back and hip.

5. Release and repeat with the left leg.

6. Finally, bring both knees to your chest and hold for 5-10 breaths.

Corpse Pose (Savasana)

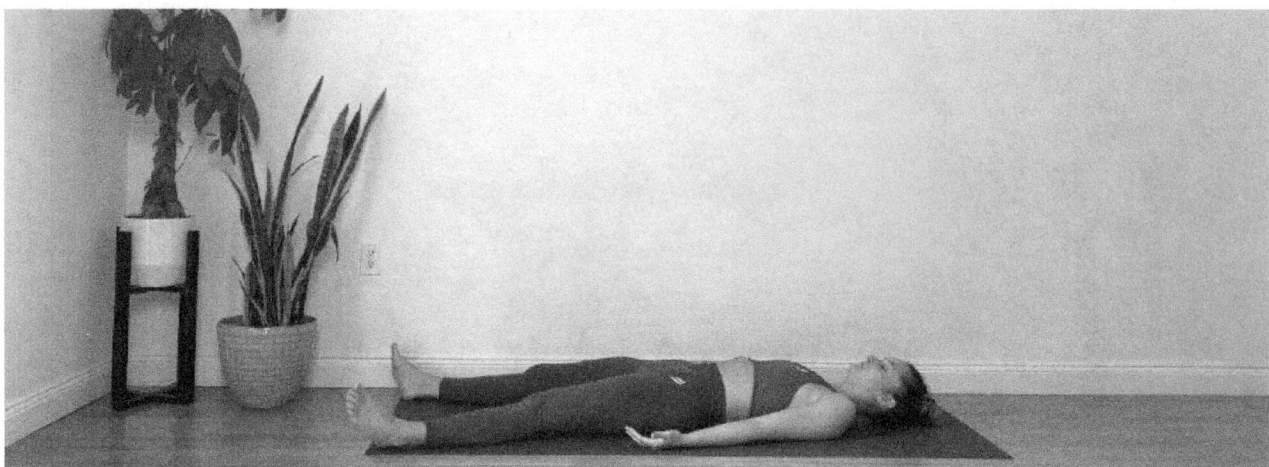

This final relaxation pose allows the body to integrate the effects of the previous exercises. It promotes deep relaxation and stress relief.

1. Lie on your back with your legs extended and arms at your sides, palms facing up.

2. Close your eyes and take a few deep breaths.

3. Allow your entire body to relax, releasing any remaining tension.

4. Focus on your breath or do a mental body scan, relaxing each part of your body.

5. Stay in this pose for 5-10 minutes, or longer if desired.

6. To exit, slowly wiggle your fingers and toes, take a deep breath, and gently roll to one side before sitting up.

Foam Rolling for Tension

Foam rolling, also known as self-myofascial release, is a form of self-massage that uses a cylindrical foam tool to apply pressure to various parts of the body. This technique targets the fascia, a connective tissue that surrounds and supports muscles, bones, and organs. Our fascia can become tight and restrictive when we experience stress, injury, or repetitive motions which leads to tension, pain, and limited mobility. Foam rolling works by applying sustained pressure to these tight areas, helping to release adhesions in the fascia and restore flexibility and range of motion.

It's very simple and effective. By using your own body weight to create pressure, you can target specific areas of tension and work them out at your own pace. This process can help improve blood circulation, reduce muscle soreness, enhance flexibility, and even aid in recovery from workouts.

Types of Foam Rollers for Tension Release

The type of roller you choose impacts your experience and the results you get. These are the various kinds of foam rollers you can use: Here's an overview of common types:

1. **Smooth, Soft Density Rollers:**
   - Best for: Beginners or those with high sensitivity to pressure
   - Features: Uniform, smooth surface with less firm foam
   - Benefits: Gentler on muscles, good for overall body rolling
   - Drawback: May not provide enough pressure for very tight areas

2. **Textured or Grid Rollers:**
   - Best for: Intermediate to advanced users, targeting specific tension points
   - Features: Surface with ridges, knobs, or grid patterns
   - Benefits: Can reach deeper into muscle tissue, good for working out knots
   - Drawback: May be too intense for beginners or sensitive areas

3. **Firm Density Rollers:**
   - Best for: Experienced users or those needing deep tissue work
   - Features: Made of denser foam or hard plastic core
   - Benefits: Provides more intense pressure, durable
   - Drawback: Can be too intense for some users, not suitable for sensitive areas

4. **Vibrating Foam Rollers:**

- Best for: All levels, particularly good for stubborn tension
- Features: Built-in vibration mechanism
- Benefits: Vibration can help relax muscles more quickly, and may reduce discomfort
- Drawback: More expensive, requires charging or batteries

5. Half Rollers or Curved Rollers:

- Best for: Spine and neck work, or those with balance issues
- Features: Flat on one side, curved on the other
- Benefits: More stable, good for specific back exercises
- Drawback: Limited versatility compared to full rollers

When choosing a foam roller for tension release, consider your experience level, pain tolerance, and the specific areas you want to target. If you're new to foam rolling, start with a softer, smooth roller and gradually progress to firmer or textured options as you become more comfortable with the technique. It's also worth noting that many people find it beneficial to have more than one type of roller to address different needs and body areas.

Chapter 7: 5-Minute Somatic Exercises

A little progress each day adds up to big results—Satya Nani

5 Minutes is enough. The fact that it's 5 minutes and not an hour doesn't make it any less effective; this is a lesson that too many people learn the hard way. For years, the fitness world has been caught in the "go big or go home" mentality. If you can't dedicate an hour to exercise, why bother at all, right? Wrong. So very wrong.

Think about a regular Tuesday; the to-do list is a mile long, stress levels are through the roof, and the thought of squeezing in an hour-long workout seems as likely as winning the lottery. On days like these, the power of 5-minute somatic exercises truly shines. What might seem pointless at first can lead to a noticeable shift. Breathing deepens. The knot in the shoulders begins to unwind. At the end of those 5 minutes, there's a difference. It's not earth-shattering, but it's there—a sense of calm, of being more centered.

It's really actually doable; day after day, those 5 minutes can be found. Sometimes in the morning before the kids wake up, sometimes during a lunch break, and occasionally right before bed. And here's the kicker: those little pockets of mindful movement start to add up. Posture improves. Chronic pain eases. Sleep gets better. It turns out that consistency trumps intensity every single time. These bite-sized somatic exercises can become a secret weapon against stress, a daily reset button. They prove that you don't need hours of free time or fancy equipment to make a real difference in how you feel.

So, If you're reading this and thinking, "I don't have time for self-care," the truth is: yes, you do. We all do. In this chapter, we'll explore a variety of 5-minute somatic exercises that can easily weave into even the busiest of days. Remember, It's all about the small, consistent steps in the right direction. Your body (and mind) will thank you.

5-Minute Somatic Exercise Plans for Anxiety

Grounding Breath and Body Scan

1. **Standing Wall Roll Down (35 seconds):** Stand with your back to the wall, slowly roll down with breath, scanning each vertebra, feeling connection to wall, roll up mindfully.

2. **Supine Arm Circles (35 seconds):** On your back, draw slow arm circles while scanning shoulder joints, feeling the weight of your arms, coordinating with deep breaths.

3. **Lying Hip Release (35 seconds):** Lie down on your back, knees bent, let knees fall side to side while scanning hip joints and lower back, breathing into any tension.

4. **Somatic Hip Rolls (35 seconds):** Still on your back, circle hips slowly, scanning pelvic region and spine connection, matching movement to breath rhythm.

5. **Reclined Butterfly Pose (35 seconds):** Lie with your knees open wide, feet together, scan inner thighs and hip creases while breathing into the belly.

6. **Seated Side Bend (35 seconds):** Sitting tall, side bend while scanning the length of torso, ribs, and side body, breathing into each space.

7. **Somatic Scapula Mobilization (35 seconds):** On your hands and knees, mindfully move shoulder blades while scanning upper back, matching breath to movement.

8. **Supine Knee-to-Chest Pose (35 seconds):** Hug knees in, scan lower back connection to ground, breathing deeply into back body.

Tension Release Sequence

1. **Cat-Cow Flow (45 seconds):** Start on hands and knees, move between arching back while lifting chest (Cow) and rounding spine while tucking chin (Cat), synchronizing movement with breath.

2. **Neck and Shoulder Release (45 seconds):** Seated comfortably, tilt ear to shoulder, make gentle head circles, and softly open and close jaw to release facial tension.

3. **Seated Side Stretch (45 seconds):** Sit tall with legs crossed, reach one arm overhead and lean to opposite side, breathing into the stretch, switch halfway through.

4. **Child's Pose to Cobra Flow (45 seconds):** Start in Child's Pose, then slide forward into gentle Cobra, return to Child's Pose, repeat 3-4 times with breath.

5. **Bridge Rolls (45 seconds):** Lie on back with knees bent, feet flat. Slowly roll the spine up and down, one vertebra at a time, coordinating with breath.

6. **Reclined Twist (45 seconds):** On your back, hug knees to chest, then drop them to

one side while looking in the opposite direction, switch sides halfway.

7. **Final Relaxation (30 seconds):** Lie flat on your back, systematically relax each body part from toes to head, focusing on deep, calming breaths.

Mindful Movement

1. **Standing Star Reach (45 seconds):** Stand tall with feet wide, reach arms up and out like a star, then fold forward, letting arms hang between legs.

2. **Cat-Cow Pose (45 seconds):** On hands and knees, alternate between arcing and rounding your back with your breath.

3. **Thread the Needle (45 seconds):** From hands and knees, thread one arm under the other, resting your shoulder and cheek on the mat, alternate sides.

4. **Child's Pose with Side Stretch (45 seconds):** Sit back on heels in child's pose, walk fingers to right then left for gentle side stretches.

5. **Gentle Bridge Lifts (45 seconds):** Lie on back, knees bent, feet flat. Gently lift and lower hips with your breath.

6. **Final Twist (45 seconds):** Lie on back, knees bent to one side, arms open in T-shape, switch sides halfway through.

Calming Hand and Foot Focus

1. **Hand Massage (2 minutes):** Gently massage each hand, focusing on the sensation.

2. **Foot Rolls (1 minute):** Roll each foot over a small ball or just on the floor.

3. **Finger Tapping (2 minutes):** Gently tap each finger to your thumb, focusing on the rhythm and sensation.

5-Minute Somatic Exercise Plans for Stress

Breath and Spine Release

1. **Somatic Wave (35 seconds):** On your hands and knees, create undulating spinal waves from tailbone to head, synchronizing movement with deep, flowing breaths.

2. **Standing Wall Roll Down (35 seconds):** Against wall, roll down and up vertebrae by vertebra, breathing deeply into each spinal segment as you move.

3. **Somatic Sunbird Pose (35 seconds):** From hands and knees, extend opposite arm and leg, breathe into the length of spine, switch sides with each breath.

4. **Dynamic Bridge Pose (35 seconds):** Lying down, roll up and down through spine with breath, inhaling to lift, exhaling to lower, moving slowly.

5. **Seated Side Bend (35 seconds):** Cross-legged, reach overhead and bend sideways, creating space between each vertebra with breath, alternate sides.

6. **Somatic Cobra Pose (35 seconds):** Lying prone, gently lift chest with inhale, lower with exhale, focusing on articulating each vertebral segment.

7. **Reclined Spinal Twist (35 seconds):** On back, knees to one side, arms open wide, breathe into the rotation of spine, switch sides halfway.

8. **Knees to Chest Rocking (35 seconds):** Hug knees to chest, rock gently side to side, massaging spine while maintaining deep, steady breathing.

Grounding and Releasing

1. **Foot Press (1 minute):** Stand and press each part of your feet into the ground, feeling the connection.

2. **Palm Presses (1 minute):** Press palms together at the chest, varying pressure. Focus on the sensation.

3. **Standing Forward Bend (2 minutes):** Bend forward from your hips, letting your arms and head hang. Sway gently.

4. **Gentle Backbend (1 minute):** Stand, hands on lower back. Gently arch backward, focusing on the breath.

Tension Melting Sequence

1. **Somatic Tabletop Cat-Cow (45 seconds):** On your hands and knees, alternate between arching and rounding your spine with your breath, moving slowly and mindfully.

2. **Butterfly Release (45 seconds):** Sit with soles of feet together, knees wide. Gently pulse knees down while keeping spine tall, then fold forward slightly.

3. **Hip Circles (45 seconds):** Still seated, extend legs wide, hands behind you, make slow circles with your torso to release lower back.

4. **Knee to Chest Rocking (45 seconds):** Lie on your back, hug knees to chest and gently rock side to side, massaging the spine.

5. **Reclined Figure-4 (45 seconds):** On your back, cross right ankle over left thigh, thread hands behind left thigh. Switch halfway through.

6. **Reclined Spinal Twist (45 seconds):** Lie on your back, draw knees to chest, then lower them to one side while turning head in opposite direction. Switch sides.

7. **Corpse Pose with Progressive Release (30 seconds):** Lie flat, systematically releasing tension from toes to head with each exhale..

Mindful Stretching

1. **Seated Side Stretch (2 minutes):** Sit cross-legged. Raise one arm overhead, and lean to the opposite side. Alternate.

2. **Seated Twist (2 minutes):** Sit with legs extended. Bend one knee, and place the opposite elbow on the outside of the bent knee. Gently twist. Switch sides.

3. **Child's Pose (1 minute):** Kneel, sit back on your heels, and stretch your arms forward. Focus on the stretch in your back.

Energy Shift

1. **Half Moon Pose (40 seconds):** Stand on one leg, hinge forward with the other leg extended back, top arm reaching to sky, focus on a point for balance, switch sides.

2. **Warrior II Pulses (35 seconds):** Step feet wide, turn right foot out, bend knee into warrior pose, pulse gently while reaching arms long, switch halfway.

3. **Standing Tree Flow (35 seconds):** Balance on one leg, place the other foot on the inner thigh or calf, grow branches (arms) up, sway gently, switch sides.

4. **Extended Side Angle (35 seconds):** From warrior II, lower forearm to thigh, extend other arm overhead alongside ear, reaching long, switch sides.

5. **Eagle Arms with Forward Fold (35 seconds):** Cross your arms at elbows, lift them up, then fold forward with soft knees, allowing the crossed arms to hang heavy.

6. **Standing Pigeon (35 seconds):** Stand on one leg, create figure-4 with other leg, fold forward slightly for balance challenge, switch sides.

7. **Triangle Pose Flows (35 seconds):** Wide stance, reach side to side in triangle pose, moving dynamically between sides with breath.

8. **Standing Forward Bend with Shoulder Opener (30 seconds):** Forward fold, interlace hands behind back, let them fall overhead while keeping knees soft.

5-Minute Somatic Exercise Plans for Trauma

Grounding and Present-Moment Awareness Sequence

1. **Standing Wall Roll Down (35 seconds):** Stand with your back against the wall, then slowly roll down vertebrae by vertebrae, let arms and head hang heavy, then roll back up.

2. **Somatic Hip Rolls (35 seconds):** Lying on your back, knees bent, feet flat, slowly roll hips in circles, allowing natural spinal movement, reverse direction halfway through.

3. **Somatic Wave (35 seconds):** Begin on hands and knees, create wavelike motion

starting from tailbone through spine to head, flowing smoothly with breath.

4. **Dynamic Warrior I (35 seconds):** Step one foot back, lift arms up, pulse back knee down while reaching up higher, creating gentle bouncing motion, switch sides.

5. **Somatic Side Stretch (35 seconds):** Stand with your feet hip-width apart, reach one arm overhead, create gentle side body lengthening with small pulses, switch sides.

6. **Seated Side Bend (35 seconds):** Sit cross-legged, reach one arm overhead, lean to opposite side, pulse gently while breathing into rib cage, alternate sides.

7. **Somatic Scapula Mobilization (35 seconds):** On hands and knees, alternate between pressing shoulder blades together and spreading them wide, moving slowly.

8. **Supine Knee-to-Chest Pose (35 seconds):** Lie on your back, hug your knees to chest, make small circles with knees to massage lower back, reverse direction..

Breath and Movement Connection Sequence

1. **Supine Arm Circles (35 seconds):** Lying on your back, draw slow circles with arms coordinating with breath, inhale as arms rise, exhale as they lower, vary circle size.

2. **Dynamic Bridge Pose (35 seconds):** On your back, knees bent, inhale to lift hips, exhale to lower, creating flowing movement synchronized with breath.

3. **Somatic Wave (35 seconds):** From hands and knees, initiate wavelike spinal movement with breath, inhale to ripple forward, exhale to ripple back.

4. **Chair Pose with Arm Waves (35 seconds):** Bend knees into chair pose, create flowing arm movements like waves, coordinating breath with each arm motion.

5. **Standing Spinal Wave (35 seconds):** Stand with knees soft, create fluid spinal motion from head to tail, letting breath guide the wavelike movement.

6. **Somatic Chest Opener (35 seconds):** Seated or standing, expand chest with breath while drawing shoulder blades together, release with exhale.

7. **Child's Pose with Arm Walks (35 seconds):** From child's pose, walk arms forward with inhale, draw back with exhale, creating rhythmic breath pattern.

8. **Somatic Shoulder Bridge (35 seconds):** Lie on your back, knees bent, lift and lower hips with breath while focusing on articulating each vertebra.

Safe Space Visualization and Anchoring

1. **Supine Arm Circles (35 seconds):** Lying on your back, trace gentle circles with arms while imagining drawing a protective circle of light around your body, breath steady and slow.

2. **Child's Pose with Arm Walks (35 seconds):** Rest in child's pose, walk arms forward creating your safe space, imagine roots growing down with each forward reach.

3. **Reclined Butterfly Pose (35 seconds):** Let the knees fall open, relaxed, imagine a soft, protective cocoon of light surrounding you as you breathe deeply.

4. **Somatic Hip Rolls (35 seconds):** On back, knees bent, gently roll hips in circles while imagining being cradled in a safe, nurturing space.

5. **Seated Side Bend (35 seconds):** Sitting comfortably, reach arm overhead and lean side to side, imagining drawing a protective arch over your body.

6. **Somatic Scapula Mobilization (35 seconds):** On hands and knees, move your shoulder blades while imagining wings of protection folding and unfolding.

7. **Lying Hip Release (35 seconds):** On your back, let your knees fall from side to side while visualizing being held in a secure, peaceful sanctuary.

8. **Corpse Pose (35 seconds):** Lie down, fully supported by earth, imagine being enveloped in a sphere of safety and peace while breathing deeply.

Important Notes:

- Always move at your own pace and within your comfort zone.

- If any exercise feels uncomfortable or triggering, it's okay to stop or modify it.

- Remember to breathe slowly and steadily throughout each exercise.

- These exercises are meant to help you feel more present and grounded in your body.

- It's normal if emotions arise during practice; acknowledge them without judgment.

- If you're working with a therapist, consider discussing these exercises with them.

EPILOGUE

I am learning to be with what is alive in me each moment. To prioritize rest in a society that worships busyness. To slow down my life to the pace of my nervous system.

In a bustling coffee shop on a Monday morning, where cups clatter and espresso machines hiss, a woman sits quietly, eyes closed. To the casual observer, she might appear to be dozing off, but look closer; her hands are resting gently on her lap, and her breath is steady and deep. She is in deep conversation with her body.

This scene plays out in countless variations every day: the man pausing at his desk to roll his shoulders and take a deep breath before a big presentation; the teenager lying on their bed, hands on their belly, feeling the rise and fall of each breath after a stressful day at school; the elderly gentleman in the park, slowly and deliberately stretching his arms overhead, savoring the sensation of muscles awakening.

These are not grand gestures, and they won't make headlines or change the world overnight, but in each of these moments, something remarkable happens: people tune in to the wisdom of their bodies and learn the subtle language of sensation and movement.

It unfolds differently for everyone. For some, it's a gradual awakening, like slowly turning up the volume on a radio that's always been playing in the background. For others, it's a sudden revelation—a moment of "Oh, this is what it means to truly inhabit my body." There are challenges along the way, of course. Old habits of ignoring bodily signals don't disappear overnight. The pressure to keep up with the frantic pace of modern life doesn't magically vanish. But with each mindful breath, each moment of pausing to check in, a new pattern emerges.

This book isn't the end; it's an invitation to continue what you've already begun, a reminder that in the midst of life's chaos, there's always an opportunity to come home to your body, to listen to its whispers, to dance with its rhythms.

So the next time you're in a coffee shop, or at your desk, or in a park, take a moment. Close your eyes. Feel your breath. Listen to the story your body is telling. It's a story of resilience, of wisdom, of the profound aliveness that resides within us all. And it's a story that's still being written, with each mindful moment, each somatic exploration.

Here's to the continual unfolding of self-discovery through somatic awareness. May we all learn to move at the pace of our nervous systems, to rest when we need to, and to celebrate the incredible intelligence of our bodies.

EXERCISE LIST

ADDITIONAL READING

10 somatic interventions explained—integrative psychotherapy mental health blog. (n.d.). Integrative Psychotherapy & Trauma Treatment. https://integrativepsych. co/new-blog/somatic-therapy-explained-methods

Aybar, S. (2021, July 21). 4 at-home somatic therapy exercises for trauma recovery. Psych Central. https://psychcentral.com/lib/somatic-therapy-exercises-for-trauma

Babauta, L. (n.d.). How to make exercise a daily habit : Zen habits. Zenhabits.net. https://zenhabits.net/how-to-make-exercise-a-daily-habit-with-a-may-challenge/

Babuta, L. (2017, February 10). Letting go of distractions. Zen Habits. https:// zenhabits.net/distractions/

Blanton, K. (2024, February 28). Somatic stretching may be the gentle workout you've been waiting for—What to know. Prevention. https://www.prevention. com/fitness/workouts/a46993501/somatic-exercises/

Burnett-Zeigler, I., Schuette, S., Victorson, D., & Wisner, K. L. (2016). Mind–Body approaches to treating mental health symptoms among disadvantaged populations: A comprehensive review. Journal of Alternative and Complementary Medicine, 22(2), 115–124. https://doi.org/10.1089/acm.2015.0038

Burton, N. (2022, November 16). 7 somatic stretching exercises for flexibility and stress relief. DailyOM.com. https://www.dailyom.com/journal/7-somatic-stretching-exercises-for-flexibility-and-stress-relief/

Byrne, C. (2022, September 22). Somatic stretching: How it works, benefits, and getting started. Everyday Health. https://www.everydayhealth.com/fitness/what-is-somatic-stretching/

Chair cat-cow pose yoga (chair Marjaryasana Bitilasana). (2017, October 15). Tummee.com. https://www.tummee.com/yoga-poses/chair-cat-cow-pose

Conlon, K. (2021, March 25). 5 Trauma release exercises you can try at home! Cohesive Therapy NYC. https://cohesivetherapynyc.com/blog/5-trauma-release-exercises-you-can-try-at-home/

Cronkleton, E. (2019, April 9). 10 breathing techniques. Healthline. https://www. healthline.com/health/breathing-exercise

Cuncic, A. (2019). Chill out: How to use progressive muscle relaxation to quell anxiety. Verywell Mind. https://www.verywellmind.com/how-do-i-practice-progressive-muscle-relaxation-3024400

Dropping anchor; an ACT skill. (2021, September 24). Flourish Mindfully. https://www.flourishmindfully.com.au/blog/dropping-anchor

Dubois-Maahs, J. (2020, October 16). What is somatic therapy and how can it benefit you? Talkspace. https://www.talkspace.com/blog/somatic-therapy-what-is-definition-get-started-guide/

Dunbar, T. (2021, December 8). The 5 keys to unlocking consistency. Curious. https://medium.com/curious/the-5-keys-to-unlocking-consistency-c9f730c47b3b

Eleanor, M. (2022, April 25). 10 types of energy healing: Which one is right for you? LocallyWell. https://www.locallywell.com/10-types-of-energy-healing-which-one-is-right-for-you/

Extended triangle pose (utthita trikonasana). (2007, August 28). Yoga Journal. https://www.yogajournal.com/poses/extended-triangle-pose/

Fargo, S. (2020, August 26). Mindfulness body scan for gratitude. Mindfulness Exercises. https://mindfulnessexercises.com/mindfulness-body-scan-for-gratitude/

Fitzpatrick, T. (2020, October 10). Relax & release lower back pain sequence. Alignsomatics.com. https://www.alignsomatics.com/blog/relax-release-lower-back-pain-sequence

Foster, L. (2023, May 16). How to choose the right gym for you: A comprehensive guide. Educate Fitness. https://educatefitness.co.uk/how-to-choose-the-right-gym-for-you-a-comprehensive-guide/

Gallo, A. (2023, February 15). What is psychological safety? Harvard Business Review. https://hbr.org/2023/02/what-is-psychological-safety

Half moon pose with chair yoga (Ardha Chandrasana with chair) | yoga sequences, benefits, variations, and sanskrit pronunciation. (2019, September 17). Tummee. https://www.tummee.com/yoga-poses/half-moon-pose-with-chair

Headache exercise. (n.d.). Somatic Movement Center. Retrieved March 27, 2024, from https://somaticmovementcenter.com/headache-exercise/

Huang, Q., & AmaniAli Babgi. (2022). Effect of Hanna somatic education on low back and neck pain levels. Saudi Journal of Medicine and Medical Sciences, 10(3), 266–266. https://doi.org/10.4103/sjmms.sjmms_580_21

Improving your body image. (2020, May 21). National Alliance for Eating Disorders. https://www.allianceforeatingdisorders.com/5-secrets-positive-body-image/

Kristen Van Bael, Ball, M., Scarfo, J., & Emra Suleyman. (2023). Assessment of the mind-body connection: preliminary psychometric evidence for a new self-report questionnaire. BMC Psychology, 11(1). https://doi.org/10.1186/s40359-023-01302-3

Lockart, E. (2023, March 27). What is grounding and can it help improve your health? Healthline. https://www.healthline.com/health/grounding

Lynning, M., Svane, C., Westergaard, K., Bergien, S. O., Gunnersen, S. R., & Skovgaard, L. (2021). Tension and trauma releasing exercises for people with multiple sclerosis – An exploratory pilot study. Journal of Traditional and Complementary Medicine, 11(5), 383–389. https://doi.org/10.1016/j.jtcme.2021.02.003

Mcphillips, K. (2020, February 20). "Somatic exercises" stretch the stress right out of your poor, aching body. Well+Good. https://www.wellandgood.com/somatic-exercises/

Mehling, W. E., Wrubel, J., Daubenmier, J. J., Price, C. J., Kerr, C. E., Silow, T., Gopisetty, V., & Stewart, A. L. (2011). Body Awareness: a phenomenological inquiry into the common ground of mind-body therapies. Philosophy, Ethics, and Humanities in Medicine, 6(1), 6. https://doi.org/10.1186/1747-5341-6-6

Miller, A. (2018). 10 Ways to use sensory experiences to build mindfulness. Happify. https://www.happify.com/hd/use-sensory-experiences-to-build-mindfulness/

Nesci, N. (2020, March 4). 5 things everyone needs to know about energy healing. The Growth & Wellness Therapy Centre. https://www.growthwellnesstherapy.com/our-blog/5-things-everyone-needs-to-know-about-energy-healing

Oschman, J., Chevalier, G., & Brown, R. (2015). The effects of grounding (earthing) on inflammation, the immune response, wound healing, and prevention and treatment of chronic inflammatory and autoimmune diseases. Journal of Inflammation Research, 8, 83. https://doi.org/10.2147/jir.s69656

Ragdoll. (2019, May 11). Yoga 15. https://yoga15.com/pose/ragdoll/

Recovery from trauma and the mind-body connection. (2023, May 9). Newport

Institute. https://www.newportinstitute.com/resources/mental-health/the-mind-body-connection/

Scott, E. (2023, August 23). How to create a "safe space" anyplace. Verywell Mind. https://www.verywellmind.com/how-and-why-you-should-create-a-safe-space-for-yourself-3144981

Shaking meditation: The easiest way to release stress in five minutes. (2019, November 19). The Times of India. https://timesofindia.indiatimes.com/life-style/health-fitness/home-remedies/shaking-meditation-the-easiest-way-to-release-stress-in-five-minutes/articleshow/72127094.cms

Stelter, G. (2018, September 20). Trap stretches: Loosen your trapezius muscles. Healthline. https://www.healthline.com/health/fitness-exercise/trapezius-stretches

Surles, T. (2023, March 15). Exercising for better sleep: 5 reasons it works. Healthline. https://www.healthline.com/health/5-reasons-exercise-improves-sleep

Toussaint, L., Nguyen, Q. A., Roettger, C., Dixon, K., Offenbächer, M., Kohls, N., Hirsch, J., & Sirois, F. (2021). Effectiveness of progressive muscle relaxation, deep breathing, and guided imagery in promoting psychological and physiological states of relaxation. Evidence-Based Complementary and Alternative Medicine, 2021(1), 1–8. https://doi.org/10.1155/2021/5924040

Tummee.com. (2024a). Seated tree pose foot side chair yoga (Upavistha Vrksasana pada parsva chair) | yoga sequences, benefits, variations, and sanskrit pronunciation. Tummee.com. https://www.tummee.com/yoga-poses/seated-tree-pose-foot-side-chair

Tummee.com. (2024b). Seated warrior pose I chair (upavistha virabhadrasana I chair) variations - 47 variations of seated warrior pose I chair | tummee.com. Tummee. https://www.tummee.com/yoga-poses/seated-warrior-pose-i-chair/variations

Upadhayay, P. (2023, February 1). How to incorporate yoga into your daily routine. Hindustan Times. https://www.hindustantimes.com/lifestyle/health/how-to-incorporate-yoga-into-your-daily-routine-101674626859419.html

Warrior II pose (Virabhadrasana II). (2007, August 28). Yoga Journal. https://www.yogajournal.com/poses/warrior-ii-pose/

What is Utthita chaturanga dandasana? (n.d.). Yogapedia. Retrieved March 10, 2024, from https://www.yogapedia.com/definition/10670/utthita-chaturanga-dandasana

Made in the USA
Monee, IL
14 January 2025

76727027R00066